baby massage

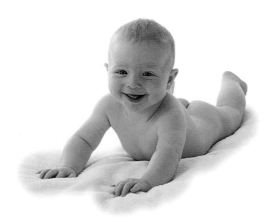

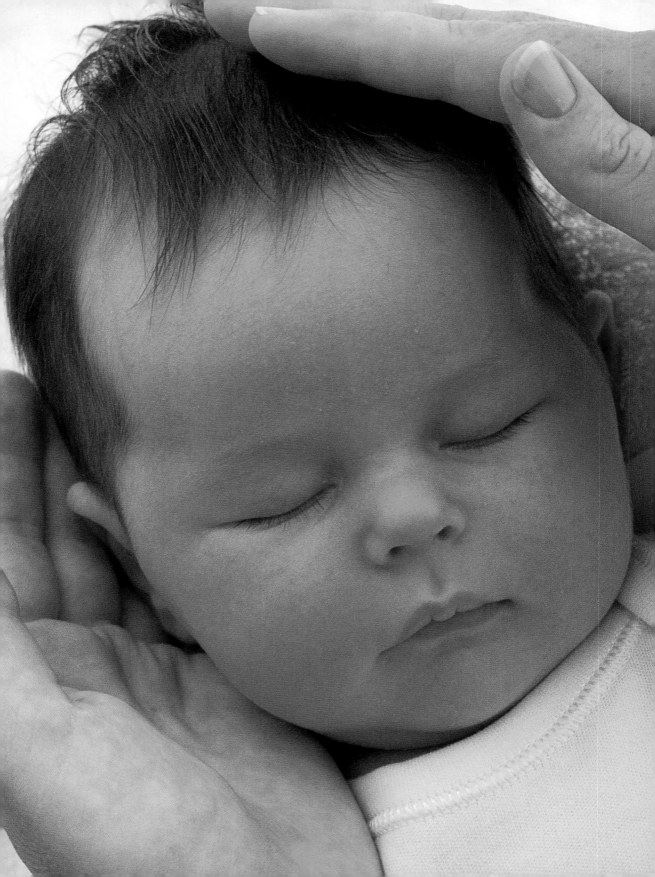

baby
massage

❖

Dr. Alan Heath & Nicki Bainbridge

Photography by Julie Fisher

LONDON, NEW YORK, MUNICH, MELBOURNE, DELHI

Revised edition
Senior editor Salima Hirani
Senior art editor Hannah Moore
North American editors Jennifer Williams, Julia Roles, Christine Heilman
DTP designers Pankaj Sharma, Balwant Singh, Karen Constanti
Production controller Sarah Sherlock
Jacket designer Katy Wall
Managing editor Anna Davidson
Managing art editors Aparna Sharma, Glenda Fisher
Art director Carole Ash
Category publisher Corinne Roberts

Original edition
Project editor Salima Hirani
Art editor Vicki Groombridge
US editor Jill Hamilton
Photographic art director Toni Kay
Production controller Joanna Bull
Managing editor Susannah Marriott
Deputy art director Carole Ash

This book is dedicated to all the children and parents who have attended our Healthy Start Clinics.

First American Edition, 2000
This edition published in 2004

Published in the United States by
DK Publishing, Inc.
375 Hudson Street
New York, New York 10014

11 10 9 8 7

016-BD148-Feb/04

A Cataloging-in-Publication record for this book is available from the Library of Congress.

ISBN 978-0-7566-0246-8

Reproduced in Singapore by Colourscan
Printed and bound in Singapore by Tien Wah Press

Discover more at
www.dk.com

IMPORTANT NOTICE
Before starting a massage on a baby or young child, refer to the warnings on page 14. If you have any doubt as to whether or not to massage any part of the child's body, seek advice from your doctor or pediatrician. Neither the authors nor the publisher can be held responsible for any damage or injury resulting from the use of baby massage.

CONTENTS

❖

❖

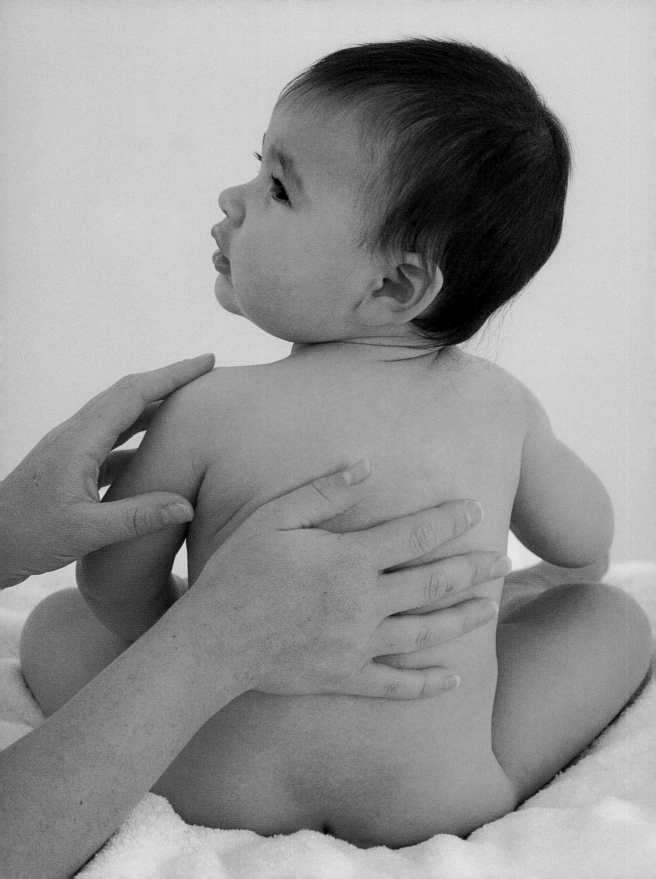

INTRODUCTION

— ❖ —

The therapeutic effects of massage on adults have been known for a long time, but only recently in the West have people realized that children can benefit from massage as well. In parts of Africa, Asia, and South and Central America, however, women have massaged their babies for centuries.

Baby massage is an integral part of the help we offer our clients at our Healthy Start Clinics. These crying, sleep, feeding, and behavior clinics were set up to advise and support parents who had difficulties with early parenting challenges. We often encountered inexperienced parents who were too nervous to touch their babies. This led to problems, since infants need plenty of positive touch to feel secure. Others had difficulty understanding their infants. If a baby cries and his parent does not know how to "make it better" (by removing the cause of distress or providing affection), the baby tends to cry more. This frustrates the parent, and a pattern is set for a downward spiral. Some of the parents who attended the clinics could not cope with an incessantly crying baby and needed to learn effective ways of coping. Others suffered from postnatal depression, a common condition that has a profoundly damaging effect on the bonding process between mother and infant; in fact, the relationship often continues to be damaged even after the condition is alleviated.

Baby massage has proven to be a practical solution to these problems. Through massaging their babies, parents gain confidence in handling them. They learn to watch and interpret their baby's reaction to touch, which sheds light on the infant's natural rhythms and on what he likes and dislikes, making it easier for the parents to understand him and, sometimes, to tolerate their own inability to soothe him. When parents enjoy watching and recognizing their child's reactions, and respond to them, the baby responds in turn, and a positive relationship develops. Parents who consulted us became visibly more affectionate toward their babies, and their children seemed happier and more self-assured. Parents reported that their babies were calmer, cried less, and slept better after they began to massage them. Parents of babies who cried a lot, usually colicky babies, claimed that even when massage did not calm their child, they felt better for trying to do something positive, which made it easier to cope. In the case of postnatally depressed mothers, there is emerging research evidence that baby massage has a beneficial role in developing the relationship between them and their babies.

These encouraging results, and the belief that all families can benefit from massage, spurred us to write this book. Massage can strengthen your baby's muscles and joints and help relieve the symptoms of some ailments that are common in the early years of life. But most importantly, it allows you to express your love for your child through touch, and helps you establish a relationship with him early on in his life.

This book is divided into four chapters. The first chapter, *Key Techniques*, demonstrates step by step all the strokes you need to give your baby a full-body massage, and gives advice on introducing massage into your baby's routine. *Everyday Care* suggests ways to incorporate additional positive touch into your daily routine, and shows how baby massage is approached in various cultures. There is also a section on how massage benefits children with special needs. *Massage for Different Age Groups* outlines the information you need to adapt your massage techniques to suit your child's developing physical and emotional needs as he grows from infancy into toddlerhood. There are also special strokes for premature babies. Finally, *Easing Common Problems* shows techniques to help alleviate the symptoms of colic, gas, constipation, teething, and dry skin, and strategies to deal with fussy crying.

The importance of touch in a child's emotional, social, and physical development is well-documented and, where relevant or illuminating, such information is highlighted in boxes throughout the book to give parents an insight into child psychology. We also reveal the results of research studies, allowing parents the opportunity to draw their own conclusions about what is right for their child.

The loving touch you share with your child through massage will enhance your relationship with him. But more than that, it will give him the security he needs to grow into a happy, confident, and emotionally secure adult.

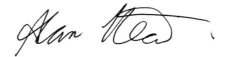

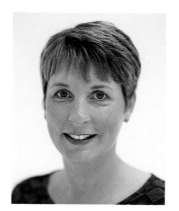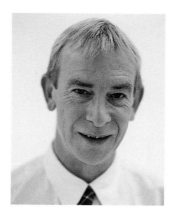

Nicki Bainbridge
RGN RHV B.Sc (Hons) ITEC
Nurse and Specialist Health Visitor

Dr. Alan Heath
BA (Hons) M.Sc Ph.D A.F.B.Ps.S
Consultant Child Psychologist

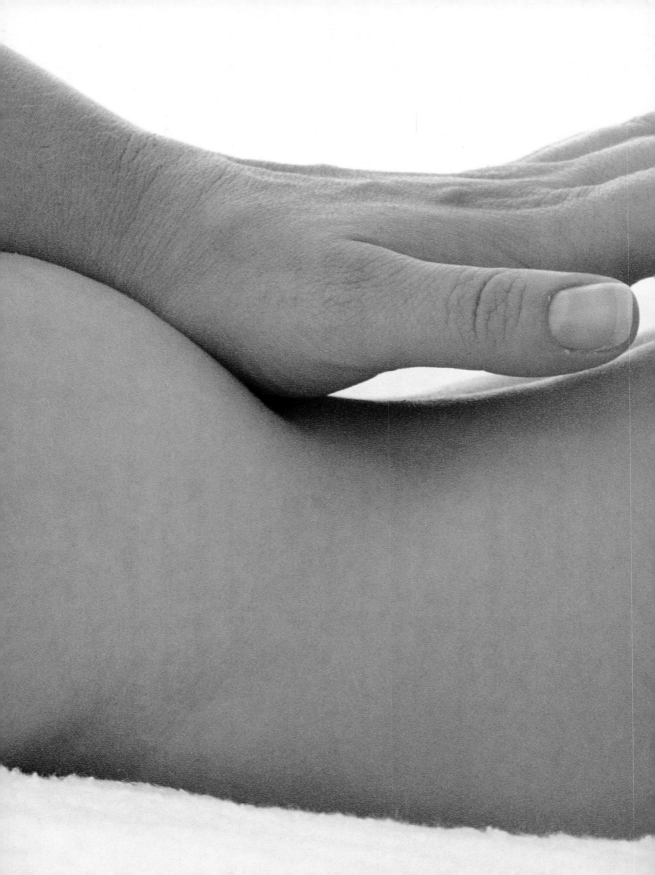

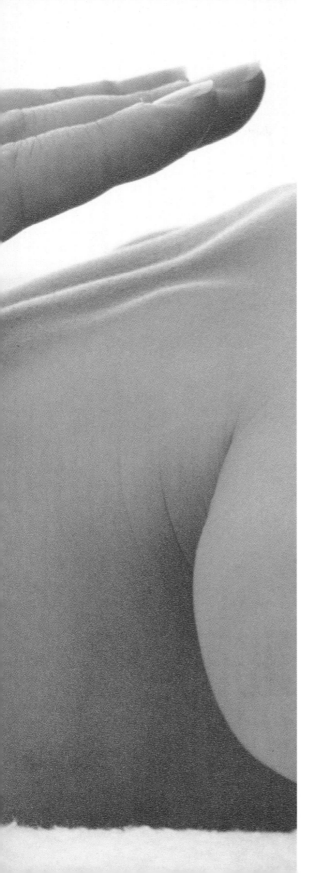

KEY TECHNIQUES

❖

MASSAGING YOUR BABY IS A WONDERFUL
THING TO DO. IT IS SO SIMPLE IN TERMS
OF TECHNIQUE, YET SO POWERFUL IN
WHAT IT CONVEYS—YOUR LOVE, YOUR
UNDERSTANDING, AND YOUR ATTENTION.
THIS SECTION INTRODUCES THE BASIC
TECHNIQUES AND MAPS OUT A HEAD-TO-
TOE MASSAGE PROGRAM FOR YOUR BABY.
APART FROM A FEW ESSENTIALS, THERE IS
NO "RIGHT" OR "WRONG" WAY TO
MASSAGE YOUR BABY. INFANT MASSAGE IS
ABOUT BEING TOGETHER AND BEING IN
TOUCH WITH EACH OTHER PHYSICALLY
AND EMOTIONALLY.

❖

WHY MASSAGE?

❖

BABY MASSAGE IS SIMPLE TO LEARN and to do. It requires little extra "equipment" and costs virtually nothing, except time. The long- and short-term benefits to infants are great, and massaging their children has a positive impact on parents, too.

BENEFITS FOR BABIES

❖ SECURITY
Positive physical contact between a parent and child makes the baby feel loved and valued. This feeling allows her self-esteem and self-confidence to develop.

❖ GENERAL WELL-BEING
Research shows that babies who are touched lovingly become ill and cry less often than those who are not. Massage can improve circulation and also boost the immune system, because it helps to move lymph fluid around the body, which clears away harmful substances. Massage may relieve pain and the symptoms of some ailments. It promotes relaxation and can help soothe a crying infant.

❖ PHYSICAL GROWTH
Massage promotes physical self-awareness, tones muscles, and makes joints more flexible. In this way, it is especially beneficial to premature babies (*see pages 62–65*), those with low birth weight, and children with special needs (*see pages 56–59*).

❖ SOCIAL SKILLS
Touching your baby teaches her about communication. Massage helps you establish a nonverbal communication with your child that enhances your early relationship with her, and therefore builds her self-esteem and sociability.

BENEFITS FOR PARENTS

❖ RELAXATION
When you massage your baby, you focus on her completely and interact with her. Parents report that they find this interaction enjoyable and relaxing.

❖ DEVELOPING SENSITIVITY
Because your baby cannot tell you if she likes a stroke or finds the pressure you apply uncomfortable, you must watch her reaction and interpret it. In this way, you learn to "read" or understand her, which improves your parenting skills.

❖ CONFIDENCE-BUILDING
Parents who are sensitive to their children tend to feel confident in their roles. Also, the physical contact of massage makes them comfortable with handling babies.

❖ PARENT–CHILD RELATIONSHIP
The nonverbal communication you share with your baby through massage sparks an interactive relationship with her that you can continue into the future. Massage can also become a regular time of intimacy between you.

RESEARCH EVIDENCE

A research study was carried out in Australia in 1992 with fathers and their babies to assess the impact of baby massage on the father–child relationship. A group of first-time fathers were shown how to massage their four-week-old babies, and asked to continue for the duration of the study. A control group of fathers who did not massage their babies was also monitored. It was found that, at 12 weeks old, babies who were massaged greeted their fathers with more eye contact, smiling, vocalizing, and touch than those in the control group. They showed more orienting responses to their fathers, and less avoidance behavior. The fathers showed greater day-to-day involvement with their infants. Baby massage allows fathers and babies to enjoy the skin-to-skin contact that mothers often experience through breastfeeding, but fathers often miss out on. By massaging their babies, fathers come to understand their child's rhythms and responses, and become more confident about handling them.

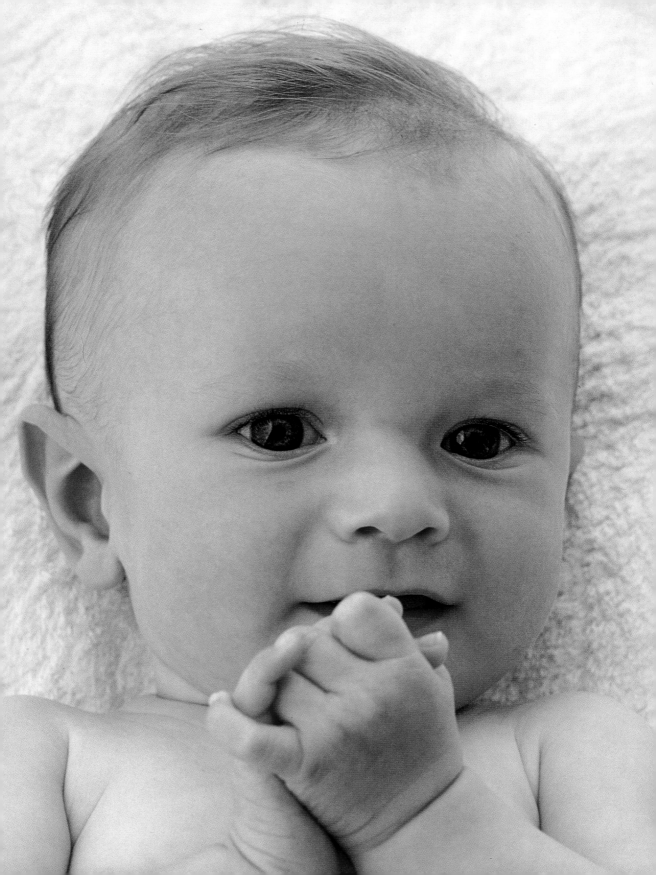

PREPARING TO MASSAGE

❖

THE BEST TIME to massage your baby is when he is awake and feeling happy. You should also be calm and relaxed because your baby will pick up on and be affected by your mood. Make sure you remove any jewelry and trim your nails to a suitable length, to avoid scratching his delicate skin. Gather everything you need around you, so that when you begin you can concentrate on the strokes, and on what your baby needs and likes, making the whole experience as soothing and pleasurable as possible for both of you.

USING OIL

WHY USE OIL?

Skin-to-skin contact promotes optimum growth and development, so undressing your baby and massaging him naked is a way of encouraging this. Oil helps your hands move over your baby's body smoothly, allowing you to make long, firm, continuous strokes without causing friction. Oil moisturizes skin, which can prevent or alleviate dryness.

WHICH OIL?

Use a natural oil, such as sunflower oil or grapeseed oil—these light, low-odor oils are easily absorbed by the skin and help to nurture it. Choose an organic variety if available. Natural oils are less likely than synthetic oils to irritate the skin. In countries where baby massage is a tradition, the oil used depends on availability. People from African and Asian cultures living in the West tend to use readily available oils that are similar to those used traditionally in their homelands, such as olive oil.

WARNINGS

❖ Oiling your baby while massaging him may make him slippery, so beware of dropping him when you lift him up after you finish the massage. Pick him up in a towel until the oil has been absorbed by the skin.

❖ If you suspect that your child may be allergic to nuts or seeds, make sure you use an oil that you know to be free of nut or seed products.

❖ Do not use essential oils (aromatherapy oils) on babies unless directed by a trained aromatherapist.

❖ Do not massage your baby if he has a fever. This is particularly important if you are unsure of the cause.

❖ If your child has any form of cancer that is being treated actively, do not massage him— you may spread the disease around the body. However, if your child is receiving palliative care, massage will be beneficial. Check with your doctor if you are unsure.

PATCH TEST

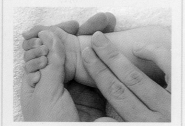

A patch test allows you to make sure your baby is not allergic to, or her skin irritated by, the oil you choose. Typical adverse reactions are a rash or a red, inflamed area.

1 Place a little oil on the inside of your baby's wrist or ankle.

2 Leave for 20–30 minutes to allow time for a severe reaction to show. To eliminate sensitivity altogether, wait for 12–24 hours.

3 If there is no irritation after this time, proceed with the massage. If irritation does occur, DO NOT use the oil.

Lay your baby on a soft towel for the massage, so that you avoid staining your clothes or carpet with oil and can pick him up in the towel after the massage

WHAT YOU NEED FOR MASSAGE

❖ A WARM ROOM
Babies lose heat quickly when uncovered and oil tends to reduce body heat, so the room must be warm enough to keep your baby comfortable. 80°F (26°C) is the ideal room temperature. If you feel warm enough in short sleeves, the room is likely to be fine for massage.

❖ THE QUIET-ALERT STATE
Massage your baby when he is in the "quiet-alert" state. This is when he is awake, alert, and bright, or when he is taking an intense interest in things around him, but remains quiet and still. He will be most receptive at this time.

❖ TIME
Allow 20–30 minutes to perform a full-body massage in the beginning. Rushing or trying to fit it in between other activities can be counterproductive because it may unsettle your baby. Once you are both familiar with the massage, you may need less time.

❖ A QUIET, CALM ATMOSPHERE
Both of you will enjoy the massage more if you are not distracted by noise from the television or radio, for example. You will "tune in" to each other more effectively, so you can be responsive to your child and notice what he likes and dislikes.

Make sure you have a cushion to sit on to help keep your back straight

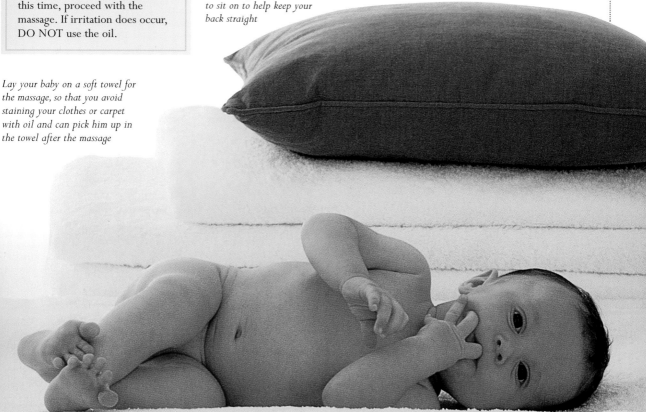

GETTING STARTED

❖

IF YOUR BABY has never been massaged, it may take her time to get used to it. Try it for three to four consecutive days initially, so you both become accustomed to the strokes. Once you feel confident and she seems comfortable with it, build it into your daily routine, or try to massage her at least three times a week. You can follow the routine in this chapter, but it is important to be guided by your baby's likes and dislikes. Use firm, reassuring strokes and make frequent eye contact with her throughout the massage.

WHEN, WHERE, AND HOW TO MASSAGE

WHEN TO MASSAGE

Massage is most effective when babies are in the quiet-alert state (see page 15). Many people like to massage after a bath in a warm room. Respond to your baby's cues. She is saying "yes" to the massage if she smiles, looks at you, and appears happy and relaxed. She is saying "no" if she cries, turns or pulls away, puts a hand over her face, or falls asleep.

WHERE TO MASSAGE

Choose a warm, quiet room where you both feel comfortable. In hot climates, massage can take place outdoors, as long as the baby is in the shade. Lay your baby on a towel on a firm surface because this promotes good posture. The floor is a good place—you can sit down to massage and there is no edge for your baby to roll off.

PRESSURE OF STROKES

Massage strokes should be firm yet gentle, deep, and slow. Always be guided by your baby. Watch for her reactions and change the pressure of your strokes accordingly. Babies find too light a touch unpleasant and irritating. Firm strokes are reassuring, but if your baby's skin reddens, reduce your pressure.

LEARNING TO RELAX

Babies absorb the tensions and anxieties of their parents, especially through physical contact. It pays for you to take time out for relaxation before beginning the massage in order for you and your baby to get the most from the experience. Clear your mind of thoughts of chores or other matters and allow yourself to give your full attention to the massage and your baby. The relaxation exercise shown here will help you unwind before you start to massage.

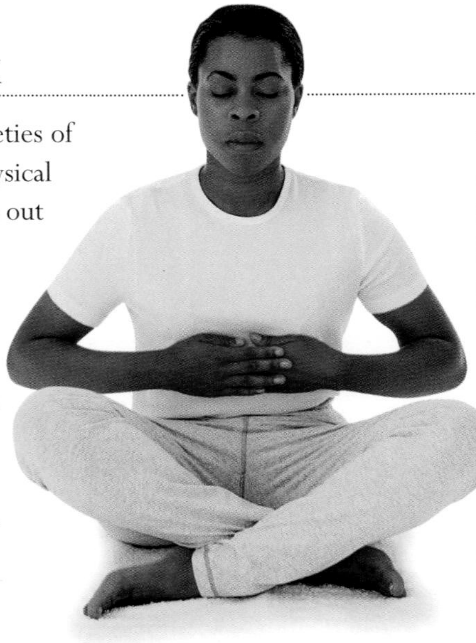

1 Clasp your fingers together and place your hands on your upper abdomen. Close your eyes and inhale deeply—you should feel your abdomen expand. Hold the breath for a few seconds, then exhale slowly.

2 Circle your shoulders backward several times, then forward. This helps relieve tension in the back, shoulders, and neck. Shake your hands vigorously.

16

CHOOSING THE RIGHT POSITION

Make sure you are comfortable when you massage. Choose a position that allows you to keep your back straight, particularly while you are leaning forward.

If you are massaging your baby on the floor, experiment with the three sitting positions shown here to find the one that suits you best.

KNEELING

Kneel on the floor with your knees resting on the towel for extra comfort. Place a cushion on your calves, under your bottom, and sit back.

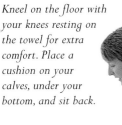

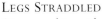

LEGS CROSSED

Sit on a cushion with your legs crossed. Place your baby directly in front of you. Lean forward and give her a few massage strokes to make sure this position is comfortable.

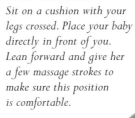

LEGS STRADDLED

Sit on a cushion with your legs outstretched on either side of your baby. You may need two cushions to keep your back straight, especially when reaching for the top of her body.

Try to keep your back straight when you lean forward to massage

Relay positive messages about communication to your baby by giving her loving looks with tender strokes—you will both enjoy this

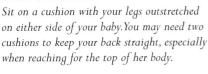

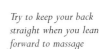

FRONT OF THE BABY

❖

Once you have warmed the room and have the oil and a towel ready, undress your baby and take off her diaper. Lay her down in front of you on her back, with her feet closest to you, ready to massage the front of her body. Dip your fingers in the oil, then rub your hands together to warm it. Each section of the massage begins with indicating to your baby which part of her body you are about to massage by placing your hands on it. Look into her eyes, smile, talk to her, and ask if you can begin. Watch for "yes" and "no" cues (*see page 16*). Responding appropriately helps her know you are sensitive to her needs. Continue to make eye contact and talk to her during the massage to reassure her.

ARMS AND HANDS

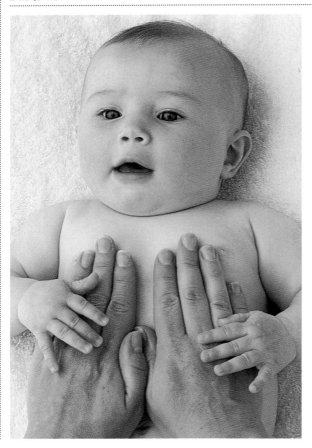

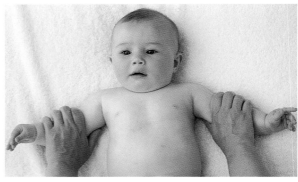

1 EFFLEURAGE STROKES ACROSS THE CHEST Place your hands on the baby's abdomen, palms facing downward and fingers pointing up the body—your fingertips should be level with the lower part of the chest. Glide both hands simultaneously up the chest toward the shoulders. Curl the fingers over the shoulders and stroke outward to take hold of the upper arms. Move directly on to step 2.

2 STROKES ALONG THE ARMS Stroke down the arms and over the hands, then pull off at the fingertips. Make sure that both your hands are working simultaneously. Initially, your baby may not straighten her arms at the elbows. As her muscles relax, you can increase the gentle "pulling" pressure of the stroke to straighten her arms. Perform steps 1 and 2 three or four times, or until the arms remain straight, even if only momentarily.

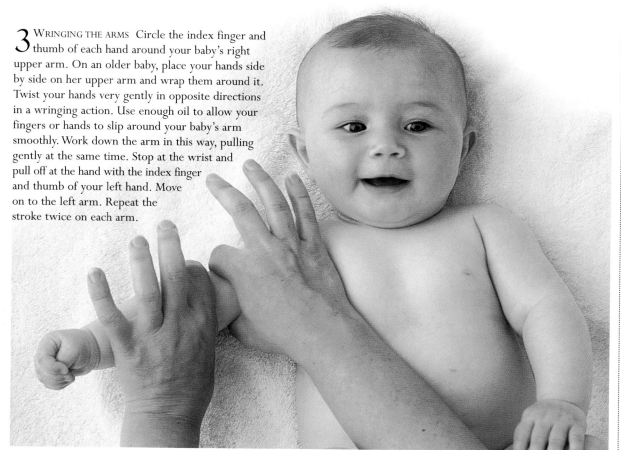

3 WRINGING THE ARMS Circle the index finger and thumb of each hand around your baby's right upper arm. On an older baby, place your hands side by side on her upper arm and wrap them around it. Twist your hands very gently in opposite directions in a wringing action. Use enough oil to allow your fingers or hands to slip around your baby's arm smoothly. Work down the arm in this way, pulling gently at the same time. Stop at the wrist and pull off at the hand with the index finger and thumb of your left hand. Move on to the left arm. Repeat the stroke twice on each arm.

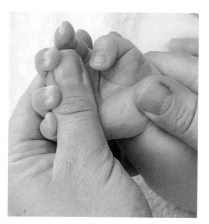

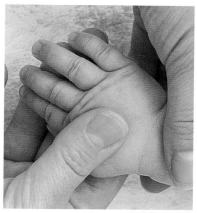

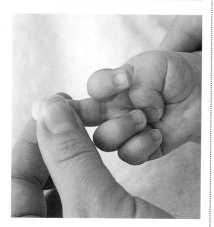

4 STRETCHING THE HANDS OPEN Support your baby's hand at the wrist with the palm facing upward. Stroke the palm from the heel of the hand to the fingertips with the thumb of your free hand, then do the same with your other thumb. Do this once more, then repeat on the other hand.

ALTERNATIVE METHOD If you find it hard to open your baby's hands as shown on the left, hold her wrist with the palm facing downward. Put your free thumb on the back of her hand near the wrist, and your fingers in her palm. Press your thumb and index finger together, and move them toward the fingers.

5 PULLING THE FINGERS Hold your baby's wrist with the palm facing upward, fingers toward you. Place your free index finger and thumb on either side of the base of the finger. Pull along the finger to the tip, squeezing lightly. Pull each digit once, then repeat on the other hand.

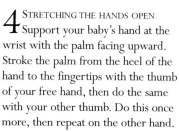

THE CHEST

CIRCLES AROUND THE NIPPLES Place the first two
fingers of each hand in the center of your baby's
chest, between the nipples. Move both sets of
fingers simultaneously, stroking upward
and outward, around the outsides of
the nipples and back to the center.
Repeat several times.

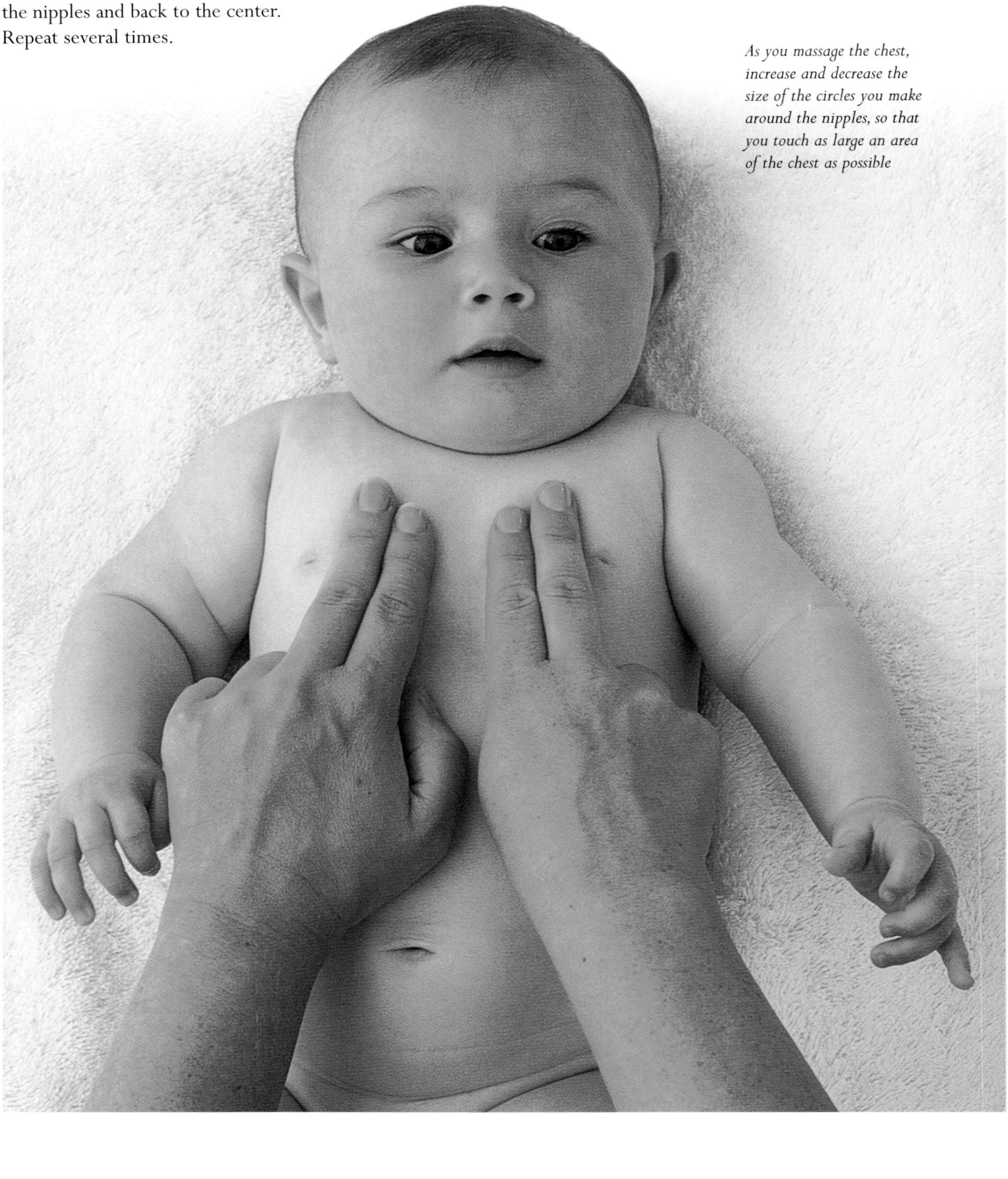

*As you massage the chest,
increase and decrease the
size of the circles you make
around the nipples, so that
you touch as large an area
of the chest as possible*

THE ABDOMEN

1 EFFLEURAGE STROKES DOWN THE ABDOMEN Place one
hand horizontally across the abdomen, just below
the chest, and stroke firmly down to the base
of the abdomen, then lift off gently. Just
before this hand loses contact with your
baby's body, place the other hand
across the top of the abdomen
as before, and stroke down.
Repeat several times,
with one hand always
in contact with your
baby's body.

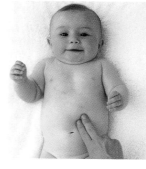

2 LITTLE CIRCLES AROUND
THE NAVEL Place the
first two fingers of one hand
next to the navel. Press
gently, making a circular
movement. Release the
pressure, slide your fingers
around the navel slightly, and
repeat. Work in a clockwise
direction, slowly spiraling
outward until you reach just
inside the right hip.

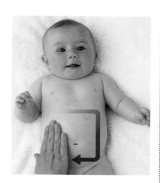

3 LARGE CIRCLES AROUND
THE ABDOMEN Starting
just inside your baby's right
hip, move the flat of your
fingers upward until they
reach the right side of the
rib cage, then across to the
same point on the left side.
Now stroke down to just
inside the left hip and across
the base of the abdomen
back to the right hip. Repeat
several times.

21

THE LEGS AND FEET

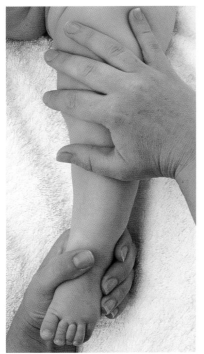

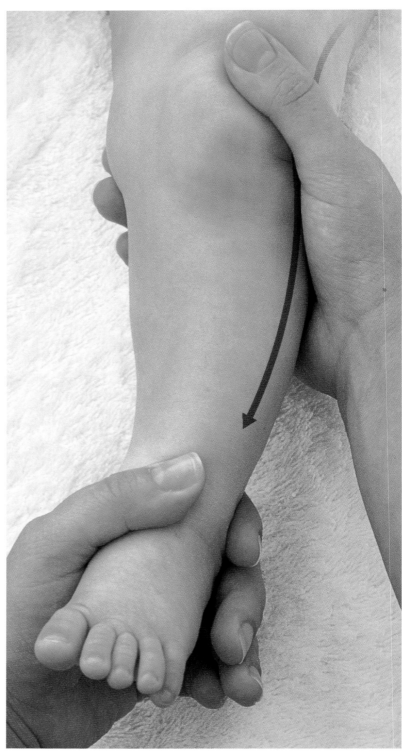

1 EFFLEURAGE STROKES ON THE UPPER LEGS Hold your baby's ankle in one hand. Place the other hand horizontally across the top of her thigh, with your fingers pointing inward. Rotate your wrist outward and fan your fingers across the thigh, around to the back of the leg, so that you are holding the thigh with your thumb on top and fingers underneath. Move directly on to step 2.

2 EFFLEURAGE STROKES ON THE LOWER LEGS Massage down the outside of the leg to the ankle. Keep holding the ankle and place your free hand back in the starting position, with fingers pointing outward. Rotate your wrist inward and stroke down, massaging the inside of the leg in the same way. Repeat steps 1 and 2 several times on each leg.

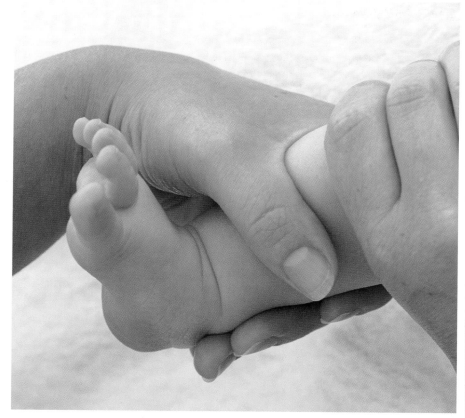

3 ▶ WRINGING THE LEGS
Place both hands next to each other on one of your baby's thighs and wrap them around it. Using light pressure, twist your hands very gently in opposite directions in a wringing action. Work down the leg, pulling gently at the same time. Stop at the ankle and pull off at the feet with your index finger and thumb. Repeat twice on each leg.

4 ▼ CIRCLES ON THE SOLES
Hold your baby's ankle in one hand, with the knee bent and the toes pointing upward. Place the thumb of your free hand at the center of the sole, near the heel. Press lightly, making a small, circular motion. Repeat the stroke up the center of the foot to the base of the toes. Do this twice on each foot.

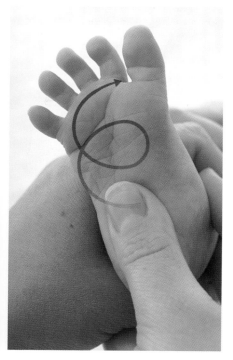

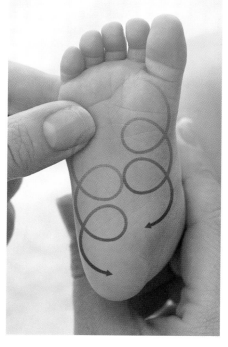

5 CIRCLES ON THE EDGES OF THE FEET Continue to hold your baby's foot in one hand, knee bent, toes pointing upward. Place your thumb on the sole directly below the little toe, and your index finger at the same position on the top of the foot. Squeeze them together, making a small, circular movement at the same time. Glide your fingers a little way down the edge of the foot and repeat the stroke. Continue in this way until you reach the heel, then use the same stroke to massage the other edge of the same foot. Do this twice on each foot.

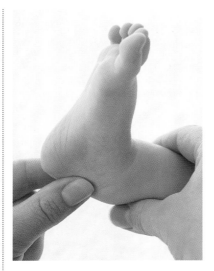

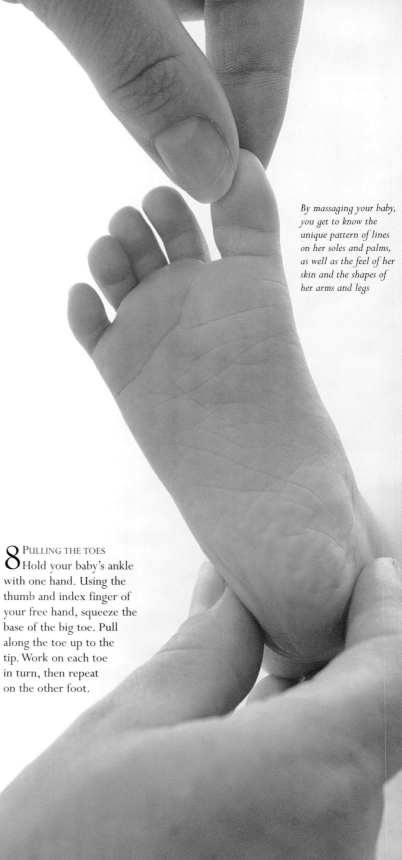

By massaging your baby, you get to know the unique pattern of lines on her soles and palms, as well as the feel of her skin and the shapes of her arms and legs

6 STROKING THE ACHILLES TENDON
Support your baby's calf in one hand, with the knee bent. Place your free index finger and thumb on either side of the ankle bone. Stroke toward the heel, squeezing gently. Do this four times, then repeat on the other foot.

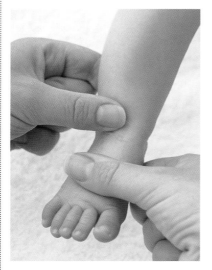

8 PULLING THE TOES
Hold your baby's ankle with one hand. Using the thumb and index finger of your free hand, squeeze the base of the big toe. Pull along the toe up to the tip. Work on each toe in turn, then repeat on the other foot.

7 MASSAGING THE TOPS OF THE FEET
Hold the ankle with one hand, making sure the knee is bent. Place the thumb of your other hand on the top of the foot near the ankle, and your index finger under the foot. Squeeze slightly, hold the pressure, pull down over the foot and off at the toes.

FINISHING STROKES ON THE FRONT

EFFLEURAGE STROKES ALONG THE BODY
Place your right hand on your baby's right
shoulder. Using your whole hand, stroke
diagonally across the chest and abdomen
to her left hip (*see below*). Continue to
stroke down the left leg to the ankle.
Do not let go of the ankle until you
have placed your left hand on your
baby's left shoulder. Now perform
the stroke on the opposite diagonal
down to her right ankle. Repeat this
twice. Make sure your strokes are
firm, and that one hand is always
in contact with your baby.

*Baby massage provides an
opportunity for you and
your baby to engage in
"conversation"—with smiles,
talking, and eye contact*

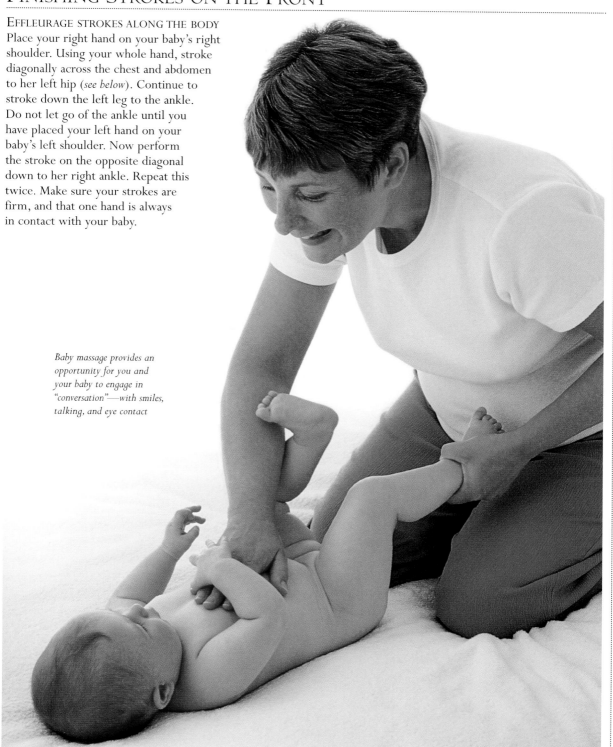

25

BACK OF THE BABY

❖

FOR THIS PART OF THE MASSAGE, position your baby on his tummy with his feet closest to you. If he is used to sleeping on his back or side, he may not like lying on his tummy, but try to encourage him to do so because it will contribute to his gross motor development. Massaging his back can be a pleasurable way of familiarizing him with this position. Initially, he may tolerate only a short stretch of time on his tummy, so perform as much of the back routine as he allows and build it up slowly. Since he will not be able to see you, talk to him and make reassuring sounds to comfort him as you massage.

THE BACK

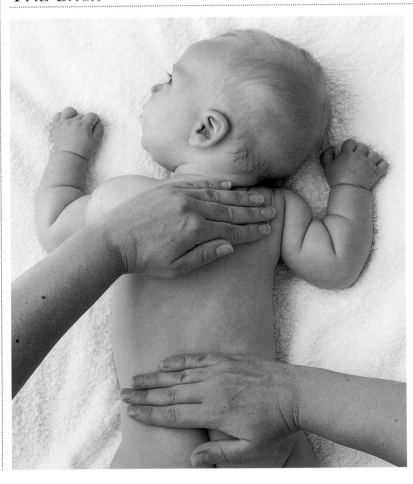

1 EFFLEURAGE STROKES DOWN THE BACK Place one hand horizontally across the top of your baby's back, just below his neck, and stroke firmly toward you. Lift your hand off when it reaches his bottom, but just before you do, place your other hand in the starting position. Stroke downward as before. Repeat these strokes several times.

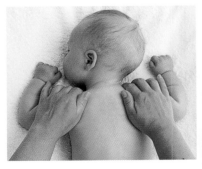

2 MASSAGING THE SHOULDERS Place one hand on either side of the neck and stroke along the shoulders toward the arms, using the whole surface of each hand. Repeat several times. Babies and parents often have identical tension spots, so if your own shoulders and neck tend to be tense, make a point of performing this stroke on your baby.

3 LITTLE CIRCLES DOWN THE SPINE Position your thumbs
on either side of your baby's spine, just below the
neck. Make small circular movements with your
thumbs while moving them down the back
toward his bottom. Make sure your
thumbs are on either side of the spine,
and not on the spine itself.

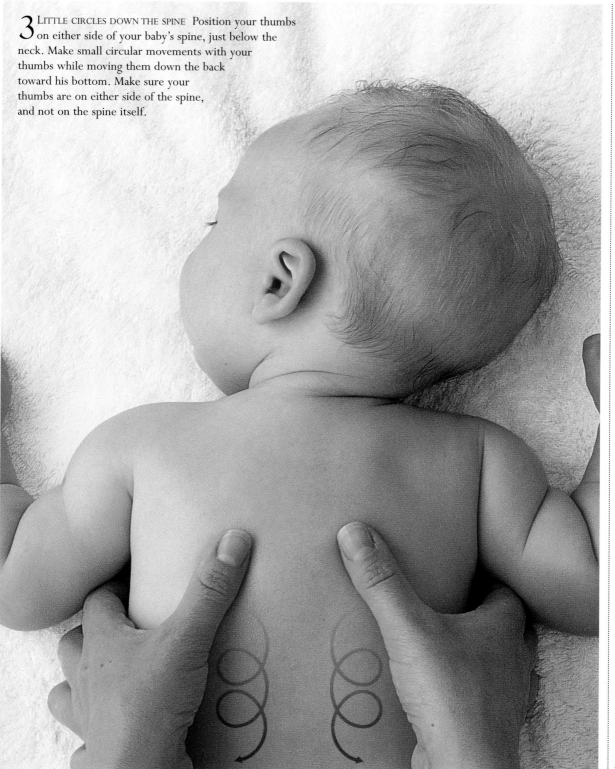

4 PULLING THE SIDES Place your hands horizontally across your baby's back (*see right*). Cross your arms and slide your right hand to his left side and your left hand to his right side. Bring your hands back to the starting position simultaneously, pulling the flesh on the sides of the torso gently toward the spine with your fingers. Make these horizontal movements several times, moving your hands up and down his back as you do so, so that you massage the sides along the whole length of the torso.

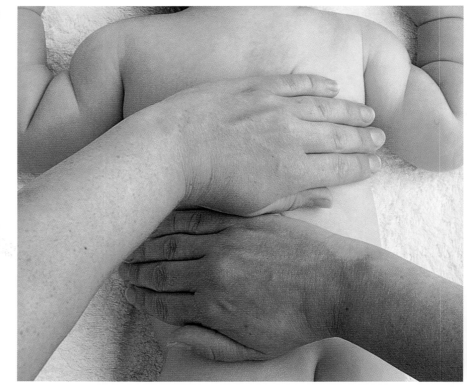

5 BIG STROKES ACROSS THE BACK AND SHOULDERS Place your hands next to each other on your baby's back, with your right hand closer to his head. Keeping your left hand in place, move your right hand to your baby's right side, then diagonally up toward and over the left shoulder. Then glide the hand down to his right hip. Now move your left hand toward his left side, then diagonally up and over his right shoulder (*see right*), and down to the left hip. Place your hands back in the starting position and repeat the stroke several times.

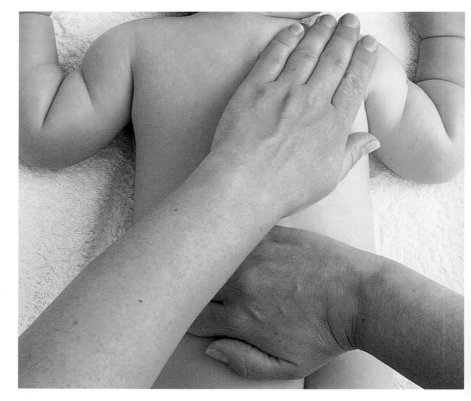

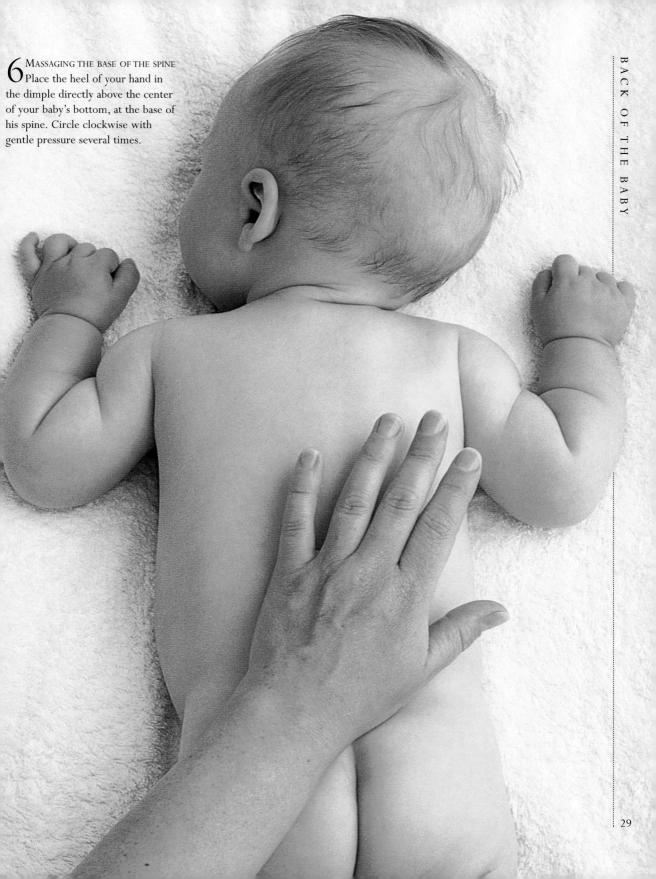

6 MASSAGING THE BASE OF THE SPINE
Place the heel of your hand in the dimple directly above the center of your baby's bottom, at the base of his spine. Circle clockwise with gentle pressure several times.

THE BOTTOM

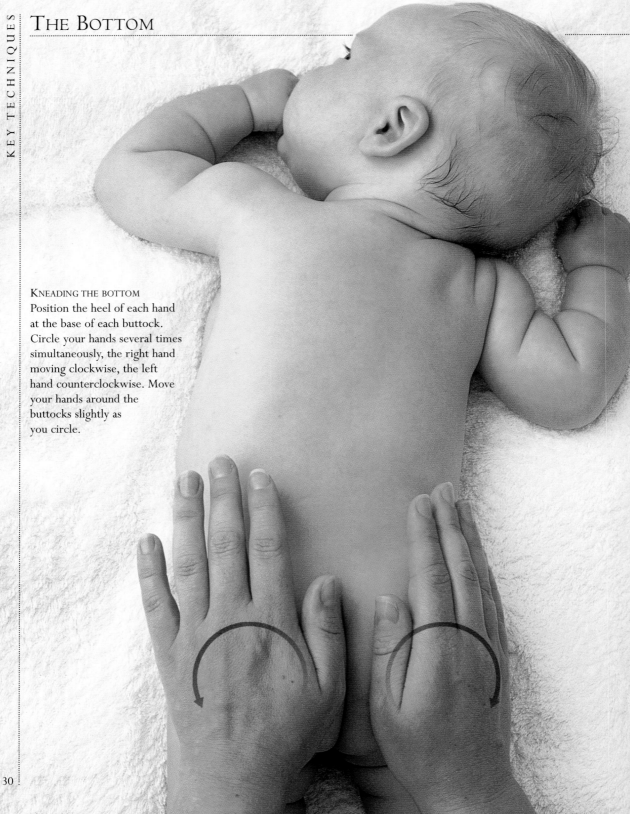

KNEADING THE BOTTOM
Position the heel of each hand
at the base of each buttock.
Circle your hands several times
simultaneously, the right hand
moving clockwise, the left
hand counterclockwise. Move
your hands around the
buttocks slightly as
you circle.

THE LEGS

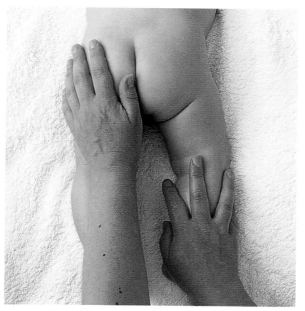

EFFLEURAGE STROKES DOWN THE LEGS Once you have finished kneading the bottom, move one hand down the leg toward the ankle in a firm, sweeping stroke. When you reach the ankle, begin the stroke on the other leg using your other hand. One hand should always stay in contact with your baby. Repeat several times.

FINISHING STROKES ON THE BACK

EFFLEURAGE STROKES DOWN THE BODY Place your left hand on your baby's right shoulder. Using the whole surface of your hand, stroke diagonally down the back, over the left buttock, and down the left leg to the foot. As you reach the foot, place your right hand on your baby's left shoulder (*see below*) and stroke diagonally down the body to the right foot. Repeat twice, using firm strokes, without losing contact with your baby's body.

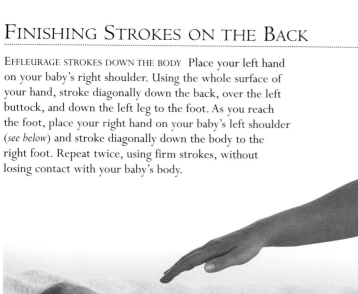

HEAD & FACE

❖

INITIALLY, BABIES TEND TO RESIST head and face massage, particularly during the first few weeks of life, especially if the delivery was long or traumatic. Try this part of the massage for three to four consecutive days. If your baby seems unhappy or cries, place still hands on his head to reassure him, then massage other parts of his body. Do this each time you massage him until he is ready for a head massage. Once babies are accustomed to these strokes, they tend to enjoy them greatly, and even more so as they get older. For this part of the massage, lay your baby on his back with his feet closest to you. Use light strokes with little or no oil.

THE HEAD

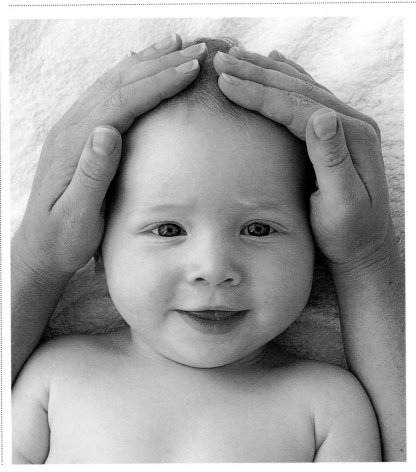

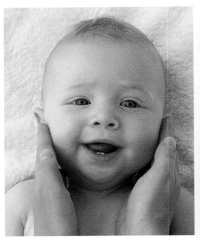

1 STROKING THE HEAD Cup your hands around your baby's head with your index fingers on his hairline. Moving your hands simultaneously, stroke backward over the crown of his head until you reach the base of the skull. Move directly on to step 2.

2 STROKING THE JAW Part your hands and bring them to the sides of his face. Stroke along the jawline with your fingers until they meet at the chin. Repeat steps 1 and 2 several times.

THE FACE

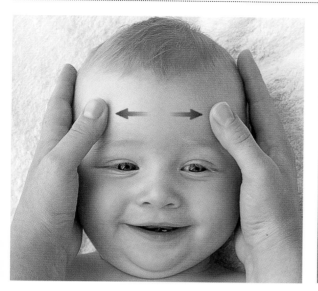

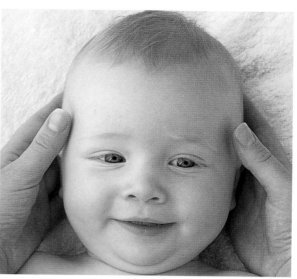

1 STRETCHING THE FOREHEAD Position your thumbs at the center of your baby's forehead, just below the hairline. Stroke each thumb outward in a straight line to the sides of the face. Repeat all the way down the forehead, as if you are drawing a series of lines with your thumbs.

2 MASSAGING THE TEMPLES On the last stroke across the forehead, place your thumbs in the center, just above the eyebrows, and gently but firmly glide them across to your baby's temples. Now make several small, circular strokes on the temples.

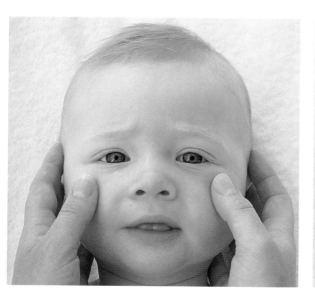

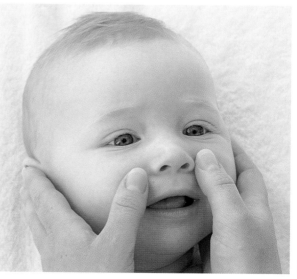

3 STROKING THE UPPER CHEEKBONES Place your thumbs on either side of the bridge of the nose. In a single flowing stroke, move each thumb simultaneously downward and outward, along the upper part of the cheekbone to the sides of the face.

4 STROKING THE LOWER CHEEKBONES Position your thumbs on either side of the bridge of the nose again, this time slightly lower down. Make a single sweeping stroke with each thumb from this position along the lower part of the cheekbone and out to the sides of the face.

33

5 CIRCLES ON THE TOP JAWLINE
Position your thumbs side by side on the dip above your baby's top lip. Pressing lightly, make small, circular movements with the thumbs. Glide each thumb outward a little and repeat. Do this along the length of the top jawline and out toward the ears.

6 CIRCLES ON THE LOWER JAWLINE
Place your thumbs side by side just below the center of the lower lip. Using light pressure, make a circular movement with each thumb, then slide them outward a little way and repeat. Do this along the lower jawline—again, toward the ears.

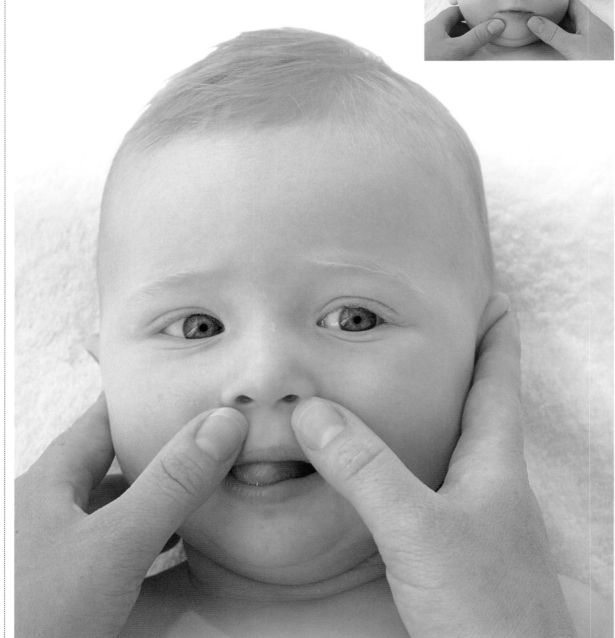

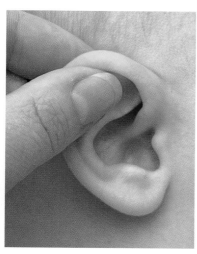

7 ◀ SQUEEZING THE EARS Hold the outer edge of the upper ear between your index finger and thumb. From this position, make small circular strokes down the outer edge of the ear to the lobe.

8 ▼ SQUEEZING THE CHIN Starting at the center of the chin, hold the flesh at the bottom of the chin between thumb and index finger and squeeze gently. Repeat along the length of the lower jawline to the ear, then on the other side of the chin. Alternatively, pinch both sides of the chin simultaneously using both hands.

9 STROKING THE HEAD Repeat the steps for the head massage on page 32 to finish the head and face massage.

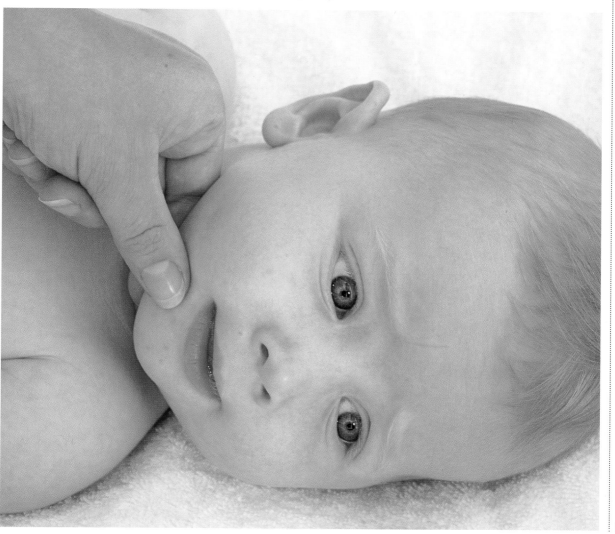

STRETCHES

❖

ONCE YOU HAVE COMPLETED the main part of the massage—on the front, back, head, and face—move on to the stretches. By now, your baby's muscles are warm and relaxed, so you can stretch the limbs and mobilize the joints safely. These stretches help to develop flexibility. For this part of the routine, lay your baby on her back with her feet toward you. Oil is not necessary. Most babies enjoy the stretches, especially when accompanied by playful noises, such as "wheeeeee!"

2 CROSSING THE ARMS Cross your baby's arms over her chest, crossing your own arms to do this. Hold the position for a few seconds. Repeat steps 1 and 2 several times. Each time you cross her arms, alternate which arm goes on top.

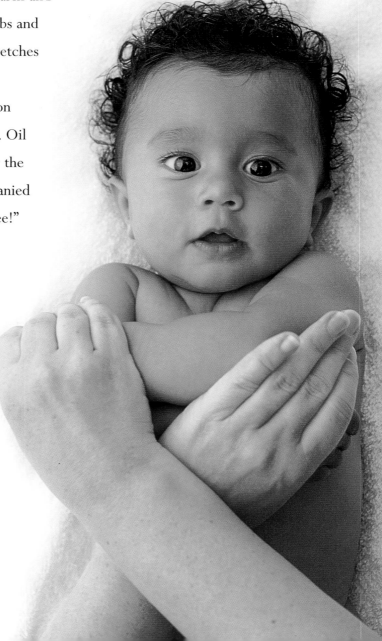

ARM STRETCHES

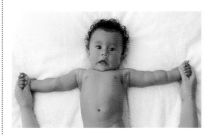

1 STRETCHING THE ARMS Hold the back of the wrists with your fingers and place your thumb in your baby's palms or on the inside of her wrists. Stretch her arms out to the sides, in line with the shoulders and at right angles to the body. Pull gently to straighten the arms. Hold for a few seconds, then move on to step 2.

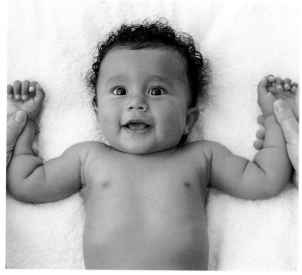

LEG STRETCHES

CROSSING THE LEGS Take hold of your baby's ankles, one in each hand. Cross them over at the lower leg. Then grasp the point where they cross with one hand and move the knees up toward the abdomen, bringing the toes near the hips. In little "bouncing" movements, press gently on the legs, easing them toward the abdomen. After a few bounces, cross the legs the other way and repeat.

3 ROTATING THE ARMS UPWARD Stretch the arms out to the sides as for step 1. Keeping the upper arms (shoulder to elbow) in position, move the hands up toward the head, so that the arms bend at the elbows. The lower arms should be at right angles to the upper arms. Make sure the arms are resting on the towel.

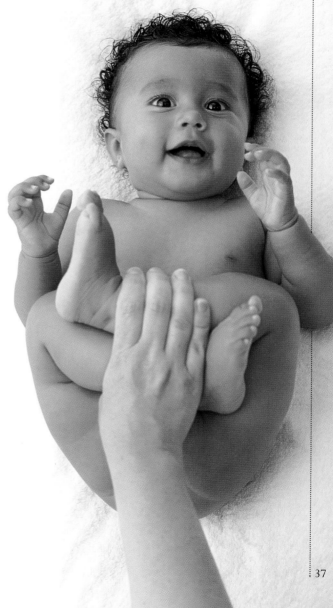

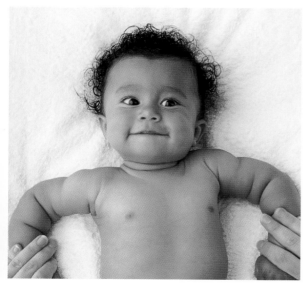

4 ROTATING THE ARMS DOWNWARD Without changing the position of the upper arms, raise the lower arms into the air so that the wrists are directly above the elbows, then bring them toward you down to the towel. The lower arms should be in line with the torso and the palms should rest on the towel. Repeat steps 3 and 4 several times.

37

ARM AND LEG STRETCH SEQUENCE

1 STRETCHING THE LIMBS Hold your baby's right wrist in your left hand, and her left ankle in your right hand. Pull both arm and leg away from the body gently at a slight angle, so the limbs form a diagonal line at each end of the torso. Hold the stretch for a few seconds, then move on to step 2.

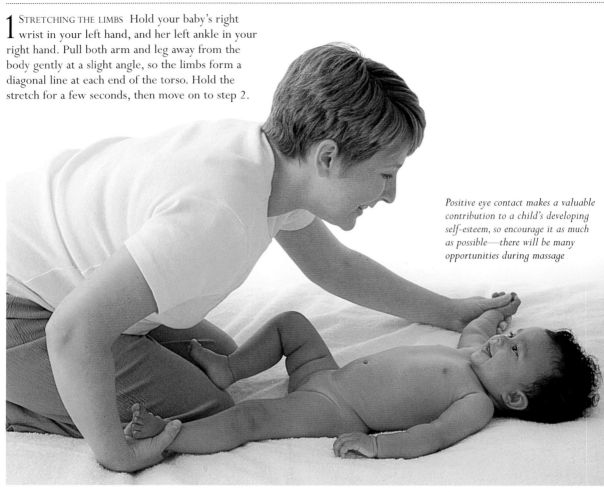

Positive eye contact makes a valuable contribution to a child's developing self-esteem, so encourage it as much as possible—there will be many opportunities during massage

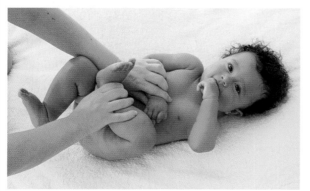

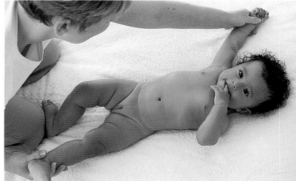

2 FOLDING IN THE LIMBS—FOOT TO HIP Bring the left foot to the right hip (leading with the heel), and the right hand to the left hip, just above the thigh. Make sure the knee is bent. Hold for a few seconds, then move on to step 3.

3 STRETCHING THE LIMBS Repeat step 1, pulling your baby's right arm and left leg gently away from her body. Again, hold the position for a few seconds, then move directly on to step 4.

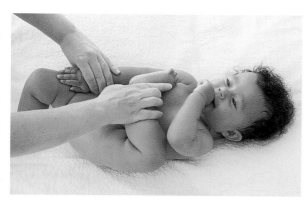

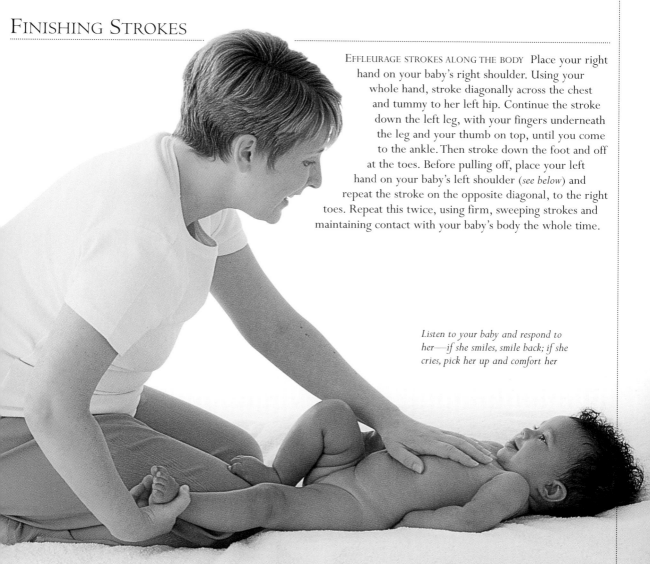

4 FOLDING IN THE LIMBS—FOOT TO SHOULDER Bring your baby's right arm straight down to the right hip, and take the left foot up to the right shoulder—again, leading with the heel. If your baby's foot does not reach the shoulder, do not force it, but take it as far as it will comfortably go. Repeat steps 1 to 4 with the same arm and leg, then twice with the alternate arm and leg.

FINISHING STROKES

EFFLEURAGE STROKES ALONG THE BODY Place your right hand on your baby's right shoulder. Using your whole hand, stroke diagonally across the chest and tummy to her left hip. Continue the stroke down the left leg, with your fingers underneath the leg and your thumb on top, until you come to the ankle. Then stroke down the foot and off at the toes. Before pulling off, place your left hand on your baby's left shoulder (*see below*) and repeat the stroke on the opposite diagonal, to the right toes. Repeat this twice, using firm, sweeping strokes and maintaining contact with your baby's body the whole time.

Listen to your baby and respond to her—if she smiles, smile back; if she cries, pick her up and comfort her

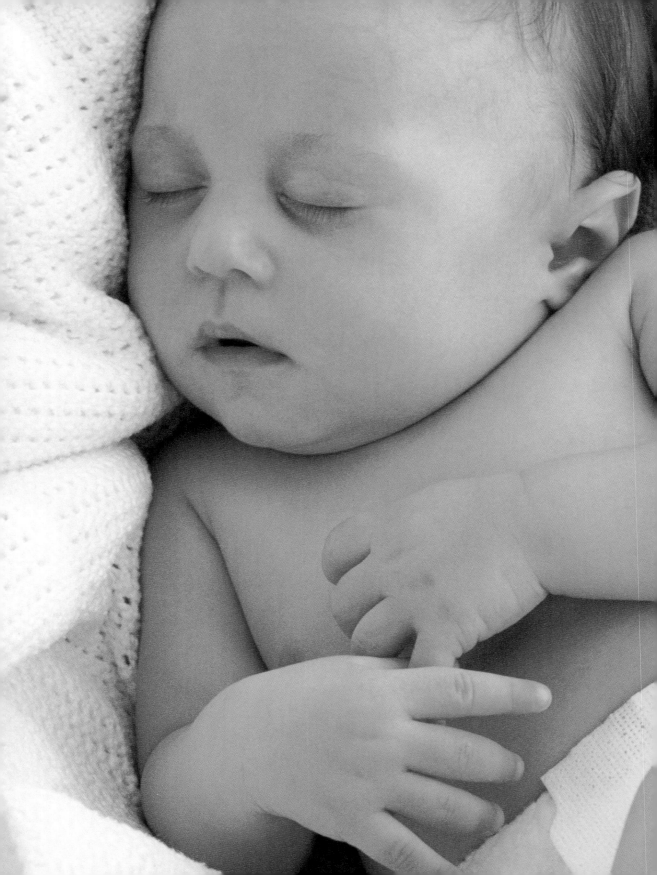

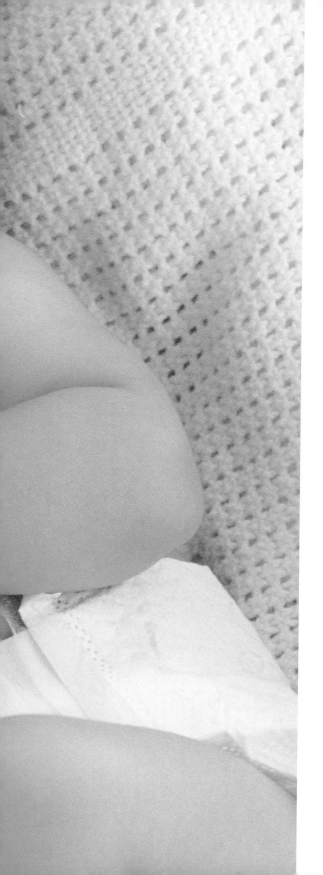

EVERYDAY CARE

❖

MASSAGE IS EASILY INCORPORATED INTO
YOUR BABY'S DAILY ROUTINE. IN FACT,
IT IS, AND HAS BEEN FOR CENTURIES, A
VALUED PART OF EVERYDAY CHILD CARE
IN MANY CULTURES, PARTICULARLY THOSE
OF AFRICA AND ASIA—AND THE
TECHNIQUES OF THESE TRADITIONS ARE
VERY INSPIRING. THERE ARE MANY WAYS
IN WHICH YOU CAN MAKE MASSAGE
AND OTHER FORMS OF LOVING TOUCH
A SPECIAL PART OF YOUR BABY
OR TODDLER'S DAY-TO-DAY LIFE,
AND IF YOUR CHILD HAS A SPECIAL
NEED, REGULAR MASSAGE CAN BE
PARTICULARLY BENEFICIAL.

❖

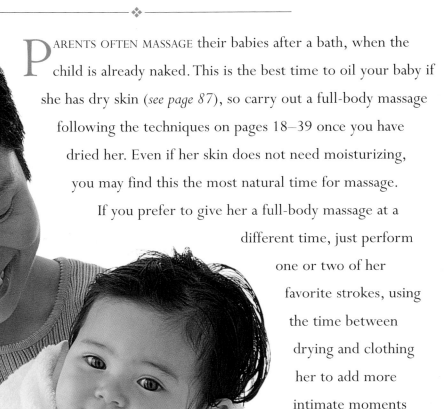

AFTER A BATH

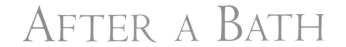

PARENTS OFTEN MASSAGE their babies after a bath, when the child is already naked. This is the best time to oil your baby if she has dry skin (*see page 87*), so carry out a full-body massage following the techniques on pages 18–39 once you have dried her. Even if her skin does not need moisturizing, you may find this the most natural time for massage.

If you prefer to give her a full-body massage at a different time, just perform one or two of her favorite strokes, using the time between drying and clothing her to add more intimate moments to your daily routine.

SWADDLING
Your baby may find it comforting to be wrapped tightly in a towel after a bath, in a fashion similar to the Chinese custom of swaddling. You can begin to massage your baby at this point, through the towel. Make firm, long strokes down her arms (see left), then cup your free hand to stroke her head (see page 47). Holding your baby with her chest to yours, make long, sweeping strokes down her back with your whole hand.

Using Effleurage Strokes

Lay your baby on a dry towel in a warm room for massage. If performing only a few strokes, try effleurage strokes on her front, back, arms (*see page 18*), and legs (*see page 22*). These allow you to touch much of her body and can also be carried out on a sitting older baby. Use oil if you like, but this is not necessary.

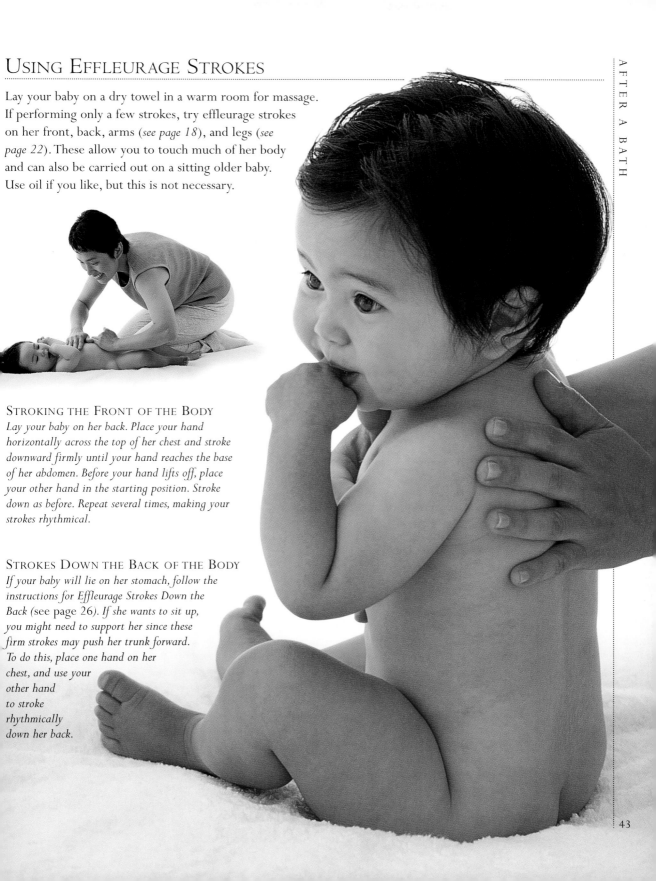

Stroking the Front of the Body
Lay your baby on her back. Place your hand horizontally across the top of her chest and stroke downward firmly until your hand reaches the base of her abdomen. Before your hand lifts off, place your other hand in the starting position. Stroke down as before. Repeat several times, making your strokes rhythmical.

Strokes Down the Back of the Body
If your baby will lie on her stomach, follow the instructions for Effleurage Strokes Down the Back (see page 26). If she wants to sit up, you might need to support her since these firm strokes may push her trunk forward. To do this, place one hand on her chest, and use your other hand to stroke rhythmically down her back.

43

DIAPER CHANGING

❖

YOU CAN MASSAGE YOUR BABY once or twice during the day when you change his diaper. Once you have cleaned him, and before you put on his diaper, stroke his tummy, legs, and feet, with or without oil. This is a good method of massaging him as he gets older and refuses to hold still for a full massage, but be prepared for the fact that he may not stay still for this either. Try the sequence for a few days, starting with just a few strokes on his tummy and legs, adding more if he tolerates them. If your baby kicks, turns over, or protests in other ways, stop— there are other ways of giving him loving touch, communicating with him, and responding to his needs (*see pages 72–73*).

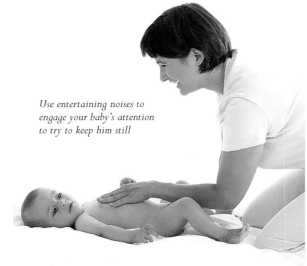

Use entertaining noises to engage your baby's attention to try to keep him still

TUMMY MASSAGE

Place your palm on your baby's abdomen. Using gentle pressure, make circular strokes in a clockwise direction with your palm, allowing your fingers to brush over his chest. Repeat several times, or for as long as your baby continues to enjoy it.

When your baby smiles at you, smile back—he will notice and enjoy it

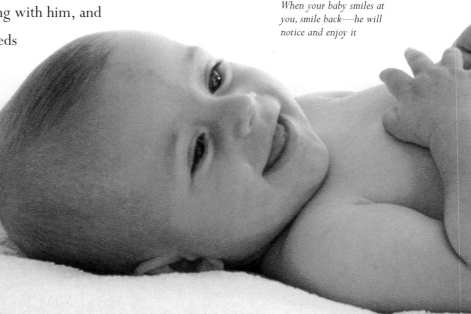

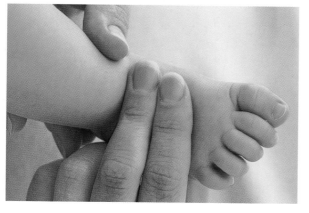

FOOT MASSAGE

Hold your baby's ankle in one hand and make sure his knee is bent. Use your free hand to hold the foot with your fingers on top and thumb underneath. Stroke firmly along the foot and pull off at the toes. Repeat several times on each foot.

LEG MASSAGE

Hold your baby's ankle in one hand. Place your free hand at the top of his thigh. Grasp the thigh, with your thumb on top and your fingers pointing upward. Stroke down his leg to his ankle. Hold the ankle with this hand and grasp the other side of his thigh in the same way as before, this time with your other hand. Stroke down the leg to massage this side of his thigh. Repeat several times on each leg.

SOOTHING TO SLEEP

❖

MANY PARENTS instinctively use massage to soothe their babies into sleep. A routine can be developed before bed- or nap-time to act as a cue for sleep. Once your baby is in her nightwear, lay her down in her crib, or cuddle her, and use strokes you know she finds particularly relaxing. Use the same sequence of strokes each time, keeping the routine short and simple. Make sure you stop before she actually falls asleep.

STROKING THE TUMMY

If your baby is lying on her back, she may enjoy a gentle tummy massage. Place your hand, palm downward, on her abdomen. Move your hand in circles in a clockwise direction, stroking her with your fingers and the entire surface of your palm. Keep the pressure very light, reducing it gently as she becomes more relaxed and sleepy, until you are hardly touching her at all.

STROKING THE HEAD AND FACE

If you are holding and cuddling your baby while she falls asleep, massage her head and face gently. Using the back of one of your fingers, stroke her cheek slowly and rhythmically. Look at her and talk or sing to her quietly. To stroke her head, cup it in one of your hands, with your index finger at her hairline. Now stroke backward to the base of her neck. Do this gently, and for as long as she finds it soothing.

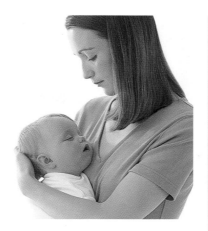

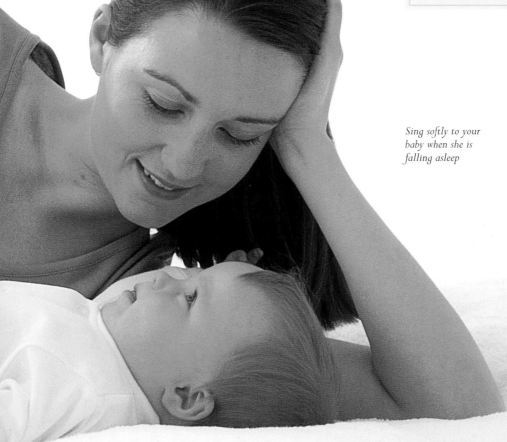

Sing softly to your baby when she is falling asleep

A CHILD PSYCHOLOGIST'S VIEW

SLEEPING ALONE Many infants fall asleep only when someone is with them. Cuddling is a vital part of parenting, but it is also important to your child's developing independence that she learns she can fall asleep alone. At about four months old, establish a sleep-time routine, such as play, bath, bedroom, breast or bottle, and crib. Take her off the breast or bottle while she is still awake but drowsy. Put her into the crib and sit with her, possibly stroking her, until she falls asleep. Over a few weeks, reduce the "help" you give, and begin to move out of the room, encouraging her to settle herself to sleep.

TODDLER PLAYTIME

❖

TODDLERS ARE FULL OF ENERGY, fascinated by life, and determined to assert their own will, so by the time your child reaches this age, you may find it hard to keep her still long enough for a full massage. Instead, try incorporating massage into playtime. Accompany strokes with games and fun noises to hold her attention for as long as possible. Devise games that involve each part of the body so that slowly, over the course of a week, you manage to massage her whole body, or most of it. But as a general rule, let your toddler's preferences guide you, and stop before she becomes distracted.

STRETCHES
Toddlers tend to enjoy dynamic movements such as stretches (see pages 36–39). They also love to count, so turn a stretch sequence into a game, with both of you counting the number of stretches you perform.

A CHILD PSYCHOLOGIST'S VIEW

ENCOURAGING SELF-CONFIDENCE Your child receives an important message when you massage her lovingly and play games with her: that you are interested in her and want to know how she feels. Assuring her in this way helps her maintain a secure attachment to you, which in turn encourages the development of her self-confidence.

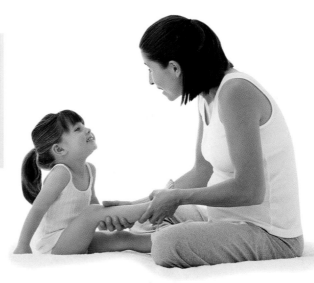

Adapt how you position your child for massage as she grows taller—if massaging her head, face, arms, or chest, bring her legs on to your lap so you can reach these areas

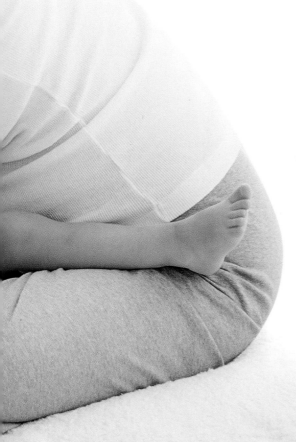

PLAYING WITH THE LEGS AND FEET

Try to adapt the strokes shown for the legs and feet (see pages 22–25) into a game such as "climbing up your legs" or "this little piggy." By incorporating a little suspense into the game, you may hold her attention for a little bit longer. Make sure that your toddler's legs are supported and her knees are bent.

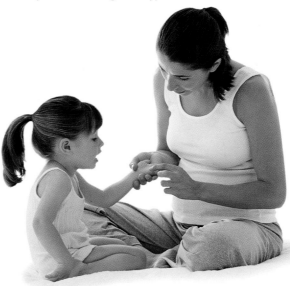

PLAYING WITH THE HANDS

Hold your child's wrist with one hand and use the thumb of your free hand to circle the palm, then pull down each of her fingers and stroke along them in turn with your index finger and thumb. Turn this into a game if you wish.

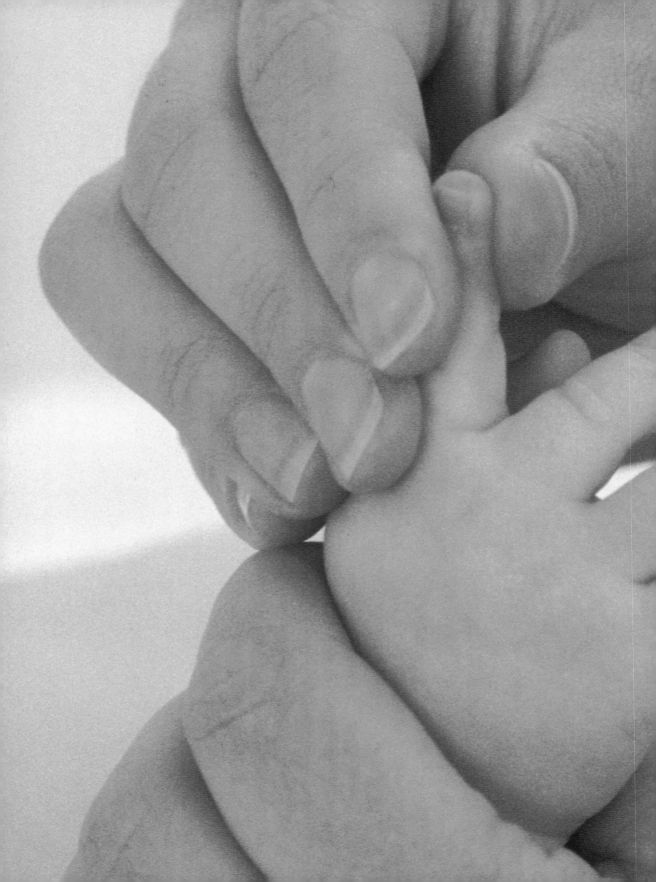

" *Massage* is something you and your baby do **together**—it's about **sharing feelings**, and even **thoughts**, on an **intimate**, unspoken level "

INDIAN MASSAGE

❖

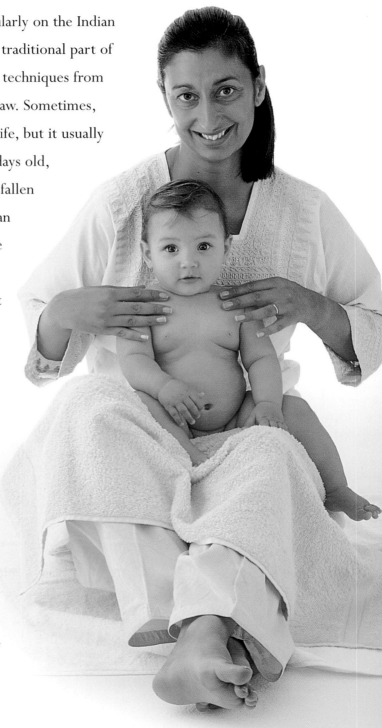

IN MANY ASIAN CULTURES, particularly on the Indian subcontinent, baby massage is a traditional part of day-to-day care. Mothers learn the techniques from their own mothers or mothers-in-law. Sometimes, massage begins on the first day of life, but it usually starts when the baby is about five days old, once the umbilical cord stump has fallen off, and continues until the child can walk. Traditionally the oils used are mustard-seed oil in the winter, because it is warming, and coconut oil in the summer because of its cooling properties. There is often no set routine. Mothers start on the areas their baby likes best and work toward those that are less enjoyed. Massage strokes and stretches are much like those shown in Key Techniques (*see pages 18–39*), and they have similar benefits.

An Indian mother or grandmother sits on the floor to massage her baby, with her legs outstretched and the baby on her lap

POSITIONS FOR INDIAN MASSAGE

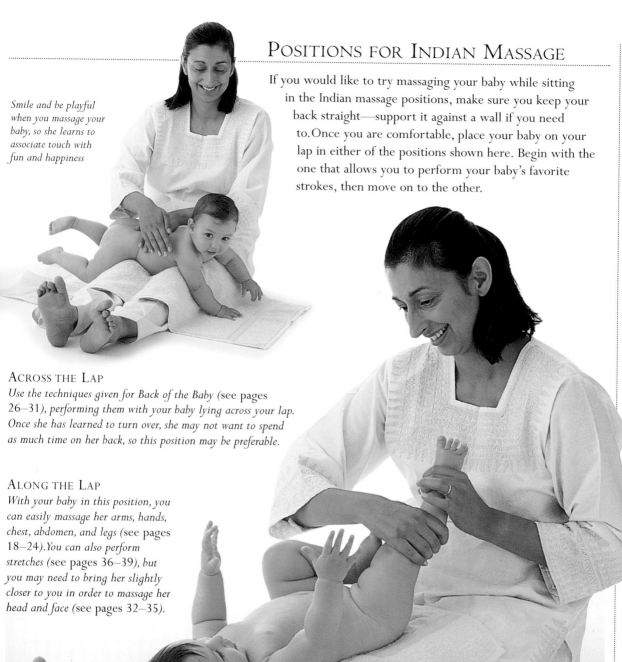

Smile and be playful when you massage your baby, so she learns to associate touch with fun and happiness

If you would like to try massaging your baby while sitting in the Indian massage positions, make sure you keep your back straight—support it against a wall if you need to. Once you are comfortable, place your baby on your lap in either of the positions shown here. Begin with the one that allows you to perform your baby's favorite strokes, then move on to the other.

ACROSS THE LAP
Use the techniques given for Back of the Baby (see pages 26–31), performing them with your baby lying across your lap. Once she has learned to turn over, she may not want to spend as much time on her back, so this position may be preferable.

ALONG THE LAP
With your baby in this position, you can easily massage her arms, hands, chest, abdomen, and legs (see pages 18–24). You can also perform stretches (see pages 36–39), but you may need to bring her slightly closer to you in order to massage her head and face (see pages 32–35).

AFRICAN MASSAGE

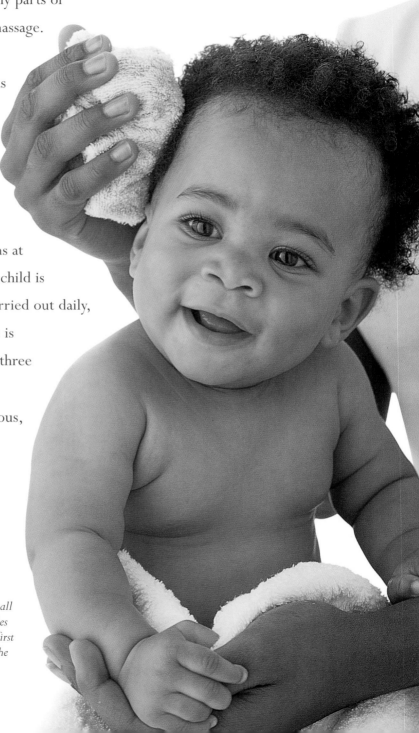

DAILY CHILD CARE in many parts of Africa includes baby massage. Techniques differ from one African culture to the next, as do the oils used. Nigerian mothers use kernel or palm oil, while in Ghana, shea butter is preferred. Massage, which traditionally takes place after a bath, begins at birth and continues until the child is three or four. At first, it is carried out daily, but as a child grows older, he is massaged less often, perhaps three or four times a week. The techniques used can be vigorous, since it is felt that strenuous movements develop strength and flexibility.

HOT PRESSES

In some parts of Africa, a baby is wrapped in a towel and placed on his mother's lap after a bath. She applies a "hot press" (simply a warmed washcloth) all over his body, in order to relax the muscles in preparation for massage. During the first few months, these are also pressed onto the head in the belief that the skull can be coaxed into an attractive shape.

NIGERIAN BABY MASSAGE

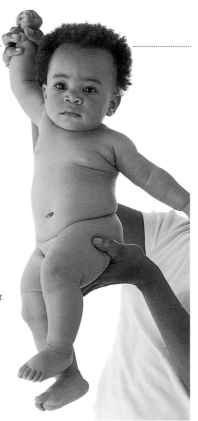

Nigerians massage their babies to help them relax and sleep well and to moisturize the skin. The mother sits in a chair with the baby on her lap. She begins with long, firm, rhythmic strokes over the arms, abdomen, legs, feet, and back. The head and face are then oiled with massage strokes. Stretches come next (*see below*); they are believed to develop strength, flexibility, and muscle tone. These are followed by the most strenuous part of the routine: dangling. The baby is held up by one arm at a time (which is believed to strengthen his arms), before being held upside-down momentarily by the ankles. Finally, he is thrown into the air and caught several times, in the belief that this develops alertness.

WARNING

Traditionally, babies are dangled by one arm, with no support. This technique, and the confidence to perform it safely, are handed down from mother to daughter. Without the guidance of an experienced demonstrator, use the adapted method shown here.

DANGLING

Sit on a chair with your baby on your lap. Place one hand under his bottom to support his weight, and hold his wrist firmly in your other hand. Stand up slowly, taking his weight in your supporting hand. Lift his arm and bring your supporting hand down marginally; his raised arm will stretch. Pull it upward gently for a few seconds, then take his weight fully in your supporting hand again. Repeat with his other arm. Always take the majority of his weight in your supporting hand, and watch his reaction to be sure he is comfortable.

STRETCHES

1 Lie your baby face-down across your lap. Take the arm farthest from your body behind his back and pull it very gently toward the center of his back, holding it straight at the elbow (*see right*). Stroke firmly from the shoulder to the wrist and pull off at the fingers.

2 Take the leg farthest from you and bend it at the knee, bringing the heel to the buttocks. Repeat several times, then stroke firmly down the legs. Change your baby's position so he faces the opposite direction and repeat on his other arm and leg.

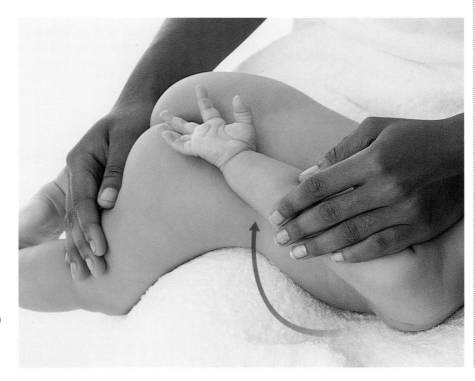

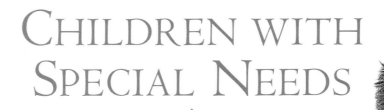

CHILDREN WITH SPECIAL NEEDS

❖

CHILDREN WITH DOWN SYNDROME or cerebral palsy often have low muscle tone, which massage can help to develop. It can also increase body-awareness; this is useful to visually impaired children, too. If your child has a special need, talk to her physiotherapist or doctor about how to massage her. Remember that she has her own rhythms that deserve respect.

MASSAGE FOR SPECIAL NEEDS

BENEFITS OF MASSAGE
Massage can:
❖ increase a child's body-awareness
❖ boost muscle tone
❖ encourage nonverbal communication between parent and child
❖ help with bonding and attachment
❖ soothe and calm children and help parents to relax
❖ allow parents to feel they are helping their child positively.

PRESSURE OF STROKES
Children with special needs often have a sensory difficulty, in that they can be either highly sensitive or insensitive to touch. They need either light or deep pressure, depending on their "sensory integration." Some children actually dislike light touch, so firm pressure is needed. If you are unsure about the pressure of your strokes, watch your baby's reaction and ask your doctor or physical therapist for advice.

CHILDREN WITH DOWN SYNDROME

If your child has Down syndrome, his muscle tone may be low. Regular full-body massages, incorporating stretches (*see pages 18–39*), help to increase muscle tone. Alternatively, he may have high muscle tone; in this case, massage can relax his muscles. If he has physical therapy, perform a quick massage before the sessions, since warming the muscles before physiotherapy may enhance the work done during a session. Some children with Down syndrome may experience hearing impairments, which massage can also help with (*see below*). In order for children with this condition to make the most of their talents and abilities, they need plenty of stimulation to respond to. Massage can be another form of stimulation that you provide for your child. It is likely that he will enjoy the massage greatly—children with Down syndrome tend to be sociable, and their cheerful and affectionate characters respond well to affectionate touch. Massage has the best results when it is something the two of you do together—a kind of touch-communication—rather than something you do to your child. Perhaps if your child has a sibling, you can encourage them to massage each other, allowing the whole family to share this form of communication. This can help improve your family relationships and make your child very happy.

CHILDREN WITH SENSORY IMPAIRMENTS

Massage helps children who are visually impaired to build a picture of the world around them, because being touched teaches them to touch, and touch helps them to explore their surroundings. A visually impaired child's body-awareness also increases through massage—she learns how long her arms and legs are, and gains a better idea of their shape. Massage can open new pathways of communication between you and your child, which will be a major source of comfort and security for her. Touch-stimulation increases the levels of responsiveness of children with sensory impairments, so massage can teach her to engage in social interaction. When you massage your child, make sure you always keep one hand on her body if she has impaired vision, and talk to her to reassure her. If your child has difficulty hearing, talk to her throughout the massage to stimulate her hearing. Tell her what you are doing, to help her link words and sounds to actions.

CHILDREN WITH CEREBRAL PALSY

Massage allows children with cerebral palsy to experience movements they cannot make alone, and increases their body-awareness. Each child's requirements are unique, so speak to your child's physical therapist to establish how massage can enhance the work done in the sessions. Regular massage enables your child to benefit frequently from movements that stimulate her physical development. Here, we show part of the routine Cordelia and her mother share before a physical therapy session.

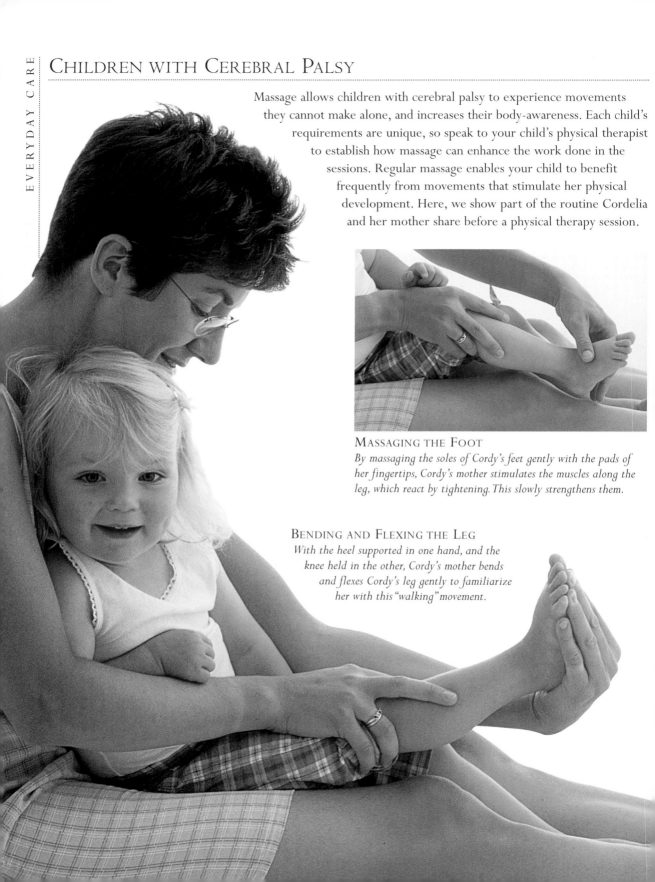

MASSAGING THE FOOT
By massaging the soles of Cordy's feet gently with the pads of her fingertips, Cordy's mother stimulates the muscles along the leg, which react by tightening. This slowly strengthens them.

BENDING AND FLEXING THE LEG
With the heel supported in one hand, and the knee held in the other, Cordy's mother bends and flexes Cordy's leg gently to familiarize her with this "walking" movement.

STRETCHING AND SITTING

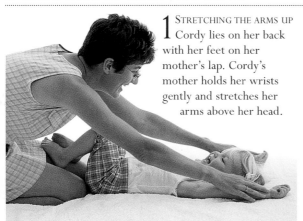

1 STRETCHING THE ARMS UP
Cordy lies on her back with her feet on her mother's lap. Cordy's mother holds her wrists gently and stretches her arms above her head.

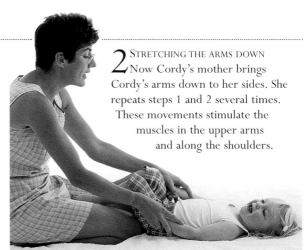

2 STRETCHING THE ARMS DOWN
Now Cordy's mother brings Cordy's arms down to her sides. She repeats steps 1 and 2 several times. These movements stimulate the muscles in the upper arms and along the shoulders.

3 SITTING UP Cordy's mother helps her come to a sitting position by pulling her arms gently. This stimulates muscles in Cordy's arms, back, and abdomen, and also in her legs, which push against her mother's lap to maintain balance as she rises up.

CASE HISTORY

"Cordy cried for weeks after the birth. Her condition was not detected immediately, so the crying was attributed to all sorts of things. When it was discovered that she had cerebral palsy, we were devastated. Her condition became noticeable when she began to move her arms and legs more and we saw that she used one side of her body more than the other. Initially, she disliked physical therapy, probably because she found it difficult, and couldn't understand what was happening to her. I think it made her dislike being touched. The physical therapist said she might relax more if we helped her do some of the movements they did together at home. We turned many of these into a game. She liked those! It did help her to relax, and now she likes to be touched."

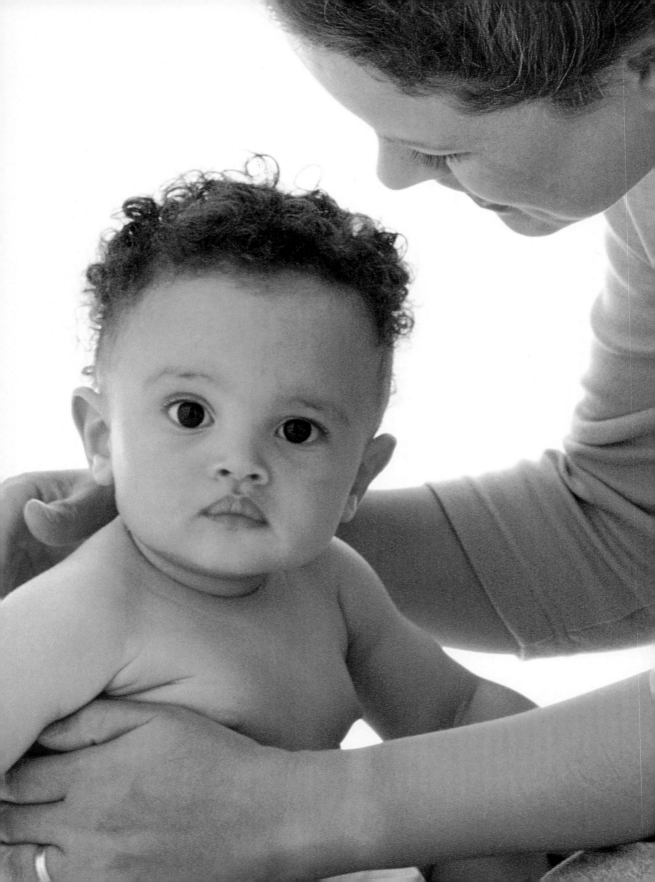

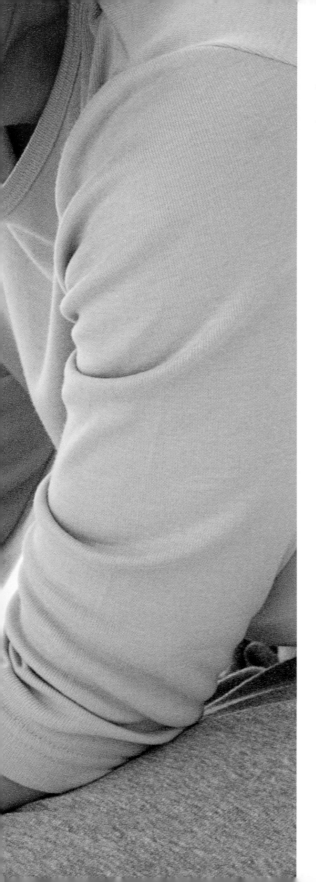

MASSAGE FOR DIFFERENT AGE GROUPS

❖

As your child develops, so do his needs, and whether he is a premature baby or a boisterous toddler, massage increases your sensitivity to him, enabling you to recognize his requirements, and decide how best to alter your approaches in response. Adapting your massage techniques, routines, and the pressure of your strokes to suit your child's changing physical and emotional needs encourages your child in each stage of development and gives him the sense that you are moving with him through his experience of life.

❖

PREMATURE BABIES

❖

HAVING A BABY who is born prematurely can be very distressing. Parents can have a range of emotions that include shock, denial, guilt, fear, anxiety, anger, and helplessness. If your baby is in an incubator, there may be little opportunity for skin-to-skin contact or eye contact. Premature babies in neonatal units are handled frequently as part of their essential medical and nursing care and often find this type of touch disturbing and distressing. Gentle touch and holding techniques are a way of giving love and comfort to a premature infant and can help parents get to know their baby.

BONDING WITH YOUR BABY

BEING THERE FOR HIM

As soon as you can, talk or sing to your baby. Babies find it reassuring to hear their parents' voices—their mother's voice in particular. It has been found that term babies turn toward their mother's voice in preference to a stranger's when only a few days old. Even if your baby appears not to respond, he will feel comforted and soothed by your voice. This is especially helpful to his well-being and the process of bonding if he is in an incubator.

STILL TOUCH

Premature babies should not be massaged initially. Instead, parents should use a technique known as still touch or resting hands (see below). This is a gentle touch, with the whole hand placed on an area of your baby's body that you feel comfortable touching, such as his back, head, arm, or leg. This touch may be the first chance you have to be close to your baby. See it as an opportunity to send your love to him. Choose a time when he is awake, calm, and alert. Place one or two hands on the chosen area and ask your baby if you can touch him before you do.

OBSERVING HIS REACTIONS

Watch your baby to gauge his reaction to this touch. He will show you, by his actions and facial expressions, whether or not he is enjoying the experience, which will help you understand what level of touch he is able to manage at this time. Keep watch for stress cues and "no" cues (see page 64). These indicate that he is becoming over-stimulated, tired, or distressed. As soon as you see any signs that tell you he has had enough, stop. You can try again the next time you notice he is awake, calm, and alert. Before using still touch or massage on your baby, talk to the nursing and medical staff about what you intend to do.

RESEARCH EVIDENCE

A research study was conducted in 1995 to identify a type of touch that parents might be able to give their premature babies in the first three weeks of life, when they may be ill and physiologically unstable.

In this study, the babies were gently touched by the adult, having still hands placed their heads and bodies for fifteen minutes a day. This type of touch seemed to have a soothing effect on these infants; they had calmer sleep, a decreased level of physical activity, and showed fewer signs of distress. The researchers reported that this touching had no adverse effects on the heart rate or oxygen saturation levels of the premature infants.

BEGINNING MASSAGE

It is important to wait until your baby is ready for massage before moving on from still touch. This may be while he is still in the hospital, or you may wait until you take him home. When you do start, begin very slowly, with just one new stroke at a time. You may wish to sit on a chair and massage your baby on your lap. Ensure that the massage strokes you use are smaller and gentler than those you might use for a full-term baby. For instance, use two or three fingers rather than the whole hand. The touch needs to be gentle but firm—too light a touch may be unpleasant and overstimulating. Before you start the massage, warm some oil in your hands. For each new body part, begin by placing your hand on that area and ask your baby if you can massage him. After each stroke, stop and observe how he reacts to it. Watch out for stress cues and "no" cues (*see page 64*). If he cries, use still hands to offer comfort and reassurance. If you respond to his cues and start a little at a time, the massage program will build up and your baby will soon anticipate and enjoy the massage.

WHEN NOT TO MASSAGE

Massage or touch techniques can be used to soothe and relax most premature infants. However, when you are using touch with your baby, it is important that you watch his reactions, especially if he is in an incubator. You should stop the massage immediately if:

❖ your baby's color changes
❖ he vomits
❖ his breathing becomes more rapid or stops
❖ his muscles become tense
❖ his pulse rate increases or becomes slow.

If any of these changes occur, inform the medical or nursing staff right away or contact your doctor.

FIRST MASSAGE
Massage your baby on your lap once he is well enough. Begin by massaging the part of his body you feel most comfortable touching and which you feel he will most enjoy. Use two or three fingers to massage a premature baby, with firm but gentle strokes. Observe your baby and gauge his reaction to each stroke.

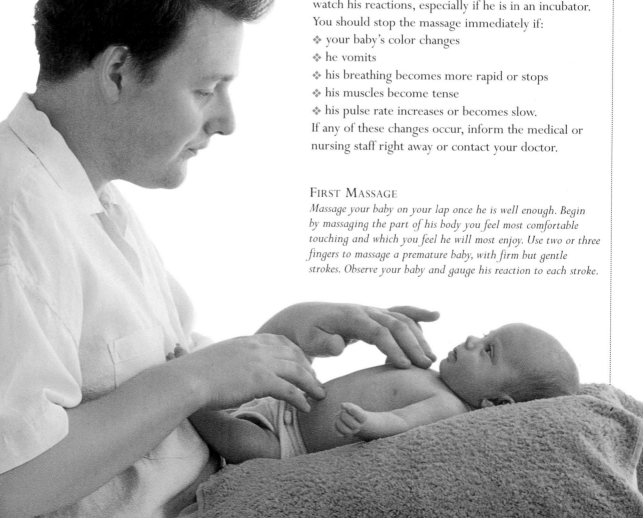

AVOIDING OVERSTIMULATION

STRESS CUES AND "NO" CUES

It is important that you do not overstimulate your premature baby with touch or massage. Observe him throughout still touch or massage to watch for when he has had enough. He will have his way of telling you that he is becoming distressed by the massage by using a stress cue, or that he wants the massage to stop by using a "no" cue, so that he can rest or sleep, for example. Signs may include:

❖ yawning
❖ sneezing
❖ hiccupping
❖ avoiding eye contact
❖ raising his hand or placing it in front of his face
❖ having an increased or decreased heart rate
❖ breathing too fast
❖ not breathing for periods of time.

Notice if your baby tends to use particular stress cues or "no" cues more than others. Learn to pick up these communications from him and respond to them. By doing so, you will improve both his well-being (by providing him with what he needs in that moment) and your relationship with him, since he will become aware that you are responsive to him and his needs.

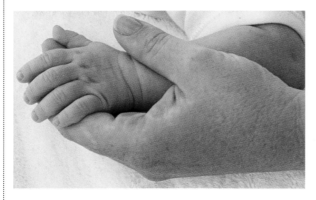

GENTLE HOLDS

Holding your baby's hand, arm, or leg is the ideal physical interaction for a premature baby. Wrap your hands carefully around the hand or limb and simply hold it for as long as your baby is happy with the touch. This gentle communication lets him know that you care for him and provides him with love and security.

LIMITING STIMULI

Although ideally it would be lovely to talk or sing to your baby, make eye contact, and touch him all at once, he may be able to deal with only one of these forms of stimulation at a time, especially during the early days or weeks. At first, limit the amount of stimulation he receives at any one time. Either talk to him *or* make eye contact with him. If he seems happy with this, it may be appropriate to move on to still touch, always watching for his reaction. In this way, progress slowly toward massage. Assess his surroundings—are his senses being overstimulated by his environment? Is the room too noisy or bright? If he is in an incubator, put a towel over part of it to limit the amount of light shining on him. Once noise is reduced to a minimum and the lighting is dimmed, he may be more able to accept interactions with you.

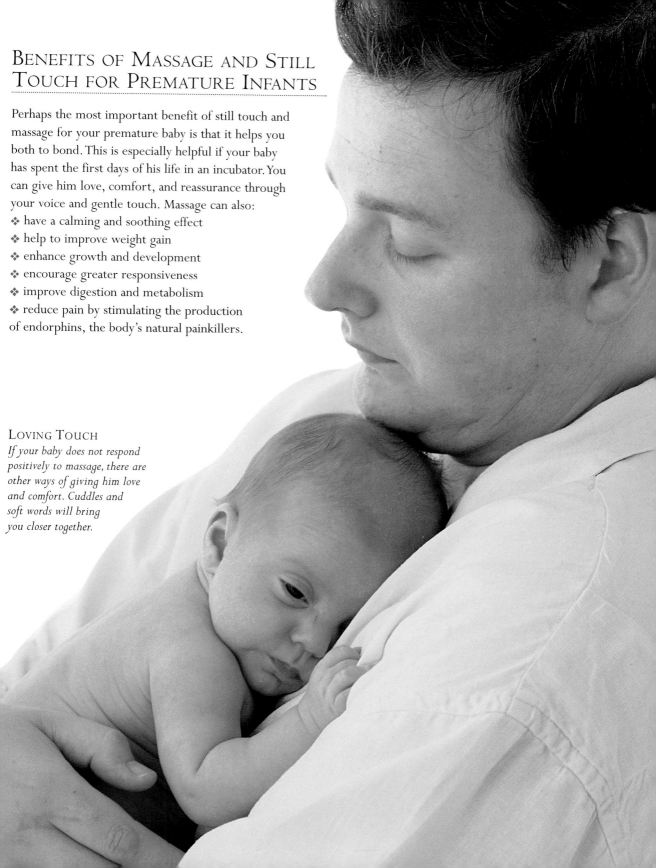

BENEFITS OF MASSAGE AND STILL TOUCH FOR PREMATURE INFANTS

Perhaps the most important benefit of still touch and massage for your premature baby is that it helps you both to bond. This is especially helpful if your baby has spent the first days of his life in an incubator. You can give him love, comfort, and reassurance through your voice and gentle touch. Massage can also:

❖ have a calming and soothing effect
❖ help to improve weight gain
❖ enhance growth and development
❖ encourage greater responsiveness
❖ improve digestion and metabolism
❖ reduce pain by stimulating the production of endorphins, the body's natural painkillers.

LOVING TOUCH
If your baby does not respond positively to massage, there are other ways of giving him love and comfort. Cuddles and soft words will bring you closer together.

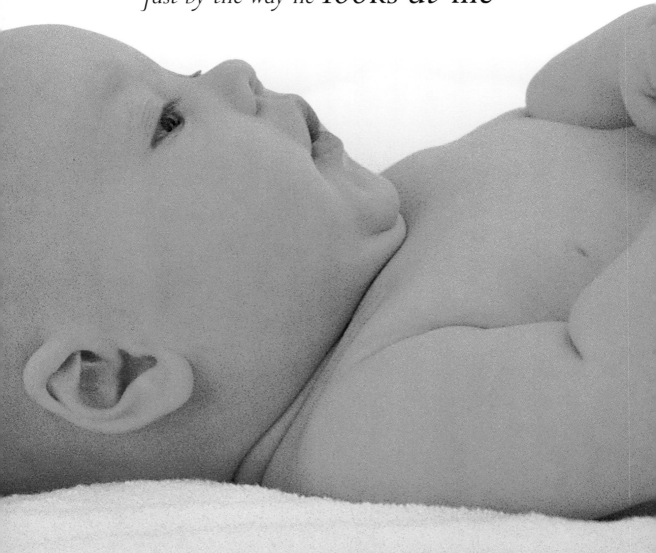

" *The* eye contact *between us is incredible.*
Sometimes **I feel** *I know exactly*
what is going through **his mind**
just by the way he **looks at me** "

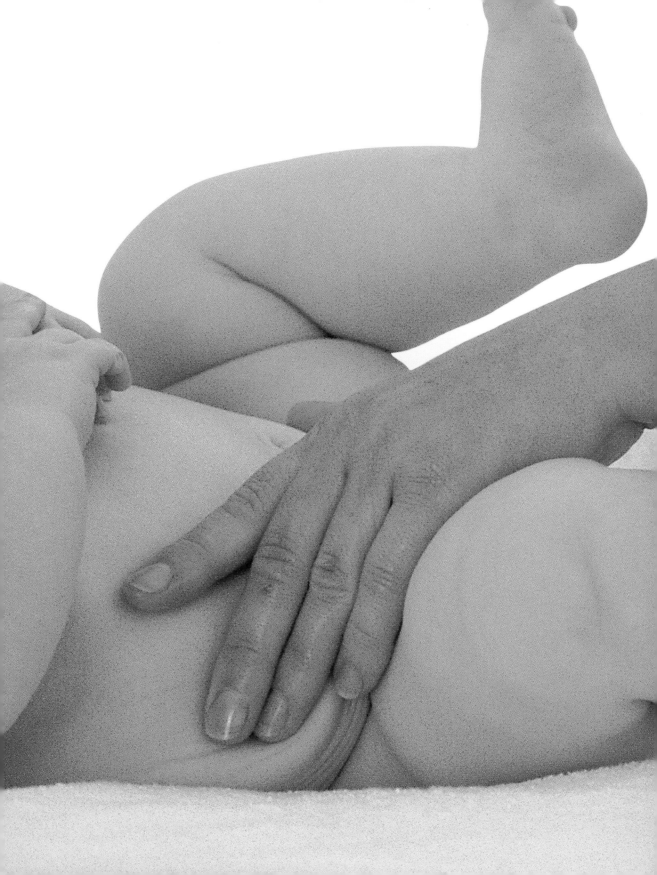

NEWBORN BABIES

MASSAGING YOUR NEWBORN BABY is a lovely way to get to know her—her expressions and reactions to different strokes, the contours of her body, the feel of her tiny fingers and toes. You will find that these special moments of loving touch are times that your baby comes to anticipate and enjoy. Massaging can also help her progress to the "quiet-alert state," in which she becomes calm, receptive,

If your newborn allows you to massage her head, take special care over the fontanelle

and seeks eye contact with you, which will create a wonderful feeling of intimacy between you. She may not smile, but you will have a sense of real closeness. This social interaction enhances your early relationship, setting strong foundations for the future.

Introducing Massage

When to Start

Baby massage can start on the day your baby is born, as happens in some cultures where infant massage is a tradition. If you feel confident and ready to begin during the first few days after the birth, then do so. Make sure you avoid touching the navel area until the umbilical cord stump has fallen off. This usually happens four to seven days after delivery.

Clothing and Seating

Some parents may initially prefer not to undress their babies for massage until both parent and child become accustomed to it. In this case, the baby can be dressed in a T-shirt or "onesie." Newborn babies, like older babies, can be massaged on the floor, but, to start with, you may find your baby prefers the

comfort and security of your lap. You can sit either on a comfortable chair, or on the floor. Place a towel over your lap to make your baby more cozy. If you choose the floor, try leaning against a wall to help you keep your back straight.

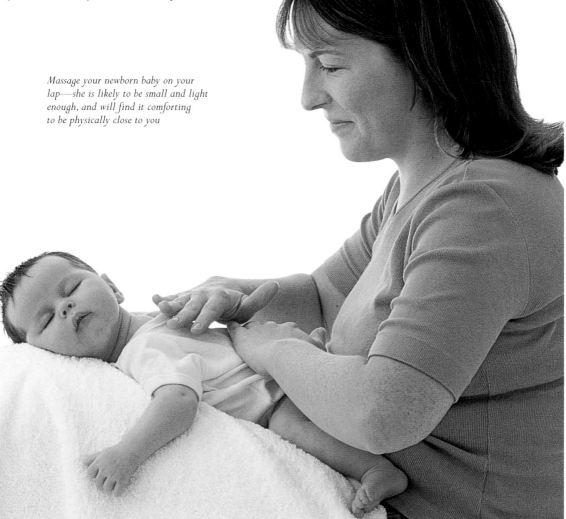

Massage your newborn baby on your lap—she is likely to be small and light enough, and will find it comforting to be physically close to you

BUILDING UP A ROUTINE

Baby massage is most beneficial for your baby when it forms part of her daily care routine. Do not worry if you find it difficult to fit it in every day. Massaging your baby as little as three times a week will still have positive results. When you introduce the massage routine, start with just a few strokes, slowly building up to a full massage over the course of three or four weeks. Begin with a short, five-minute session using long,

gliding (effleurage) strokes (*see right*). Make the strokes firm and slow. Watch your baby's reaction. She will let you know what she likes and dislikes (*see page 16*). As you both gain confidence, remove your baby's clothes and massage her using oil. Gradually add more strokes until the routine has developed into a 15–20-minute full-body massage (*see pages 18–35*), ending with stretches (*see pages 36–39*).

INCORPORATING STROKES

There are two ways of adding new strokes to your routine:

❖ Massage each part of the body—the front, back, head, and face—incorporating more strokes into each section every time until you are using all the key techniques.

❖ Start on the front of the body (*see page 18*), move on to the back (*see page 26*) and the head and face (*see page 32*), then add stretches.

LIGHT TOUCH
Initially, you may prefer to use light, delicate strokes to familiarize both you and your newborn baby with touch and massage. Use both hands in succession to make slow, light, rhythmic strokes with your fingertips on her arms and legs. Watch your baby's reaction to this stroke. Some babies prefer a firmer touch right away.

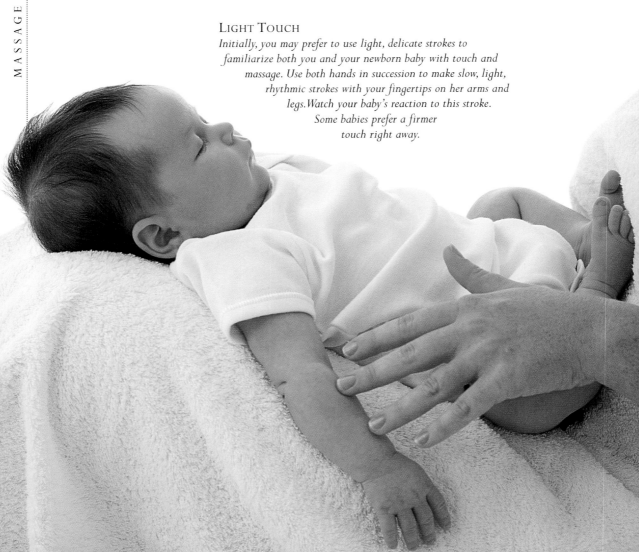

EFFLEURAGE STROKES

Babies find big, firm effleurage strokes reassuring. Use your whole palms and the flat of your fingers to stroke over your baby's abdomen (see page 21), arms, legs, and back. Ensure that one hand is always touching your baby. Before you start massaging any part of the body, place both hands on the part you intend to massage and ask your baby if you can begin. Observe her reactions to the massage constantly and respond appropriately.

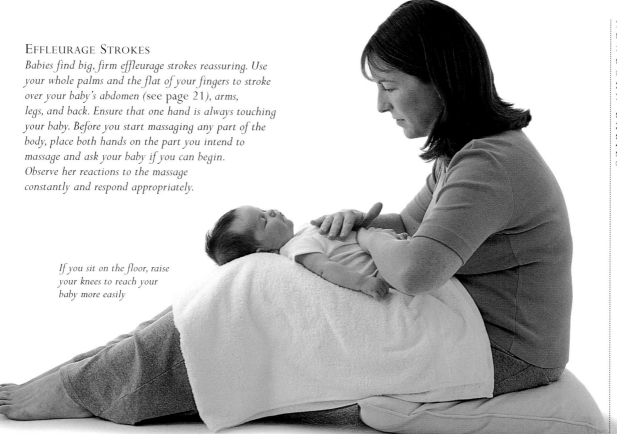

If you sit on the floor, raise your knees to reach your baby more easily

IF YOUR BABY DISLIKES IT

Some babies enjoy massage right away; others take a few days to get used to each stroke. Massaging on consecutive days will help, as will massaging her when she is in the quiet-alert state (*see page 15*). To make her feel secure, place a rolled-up towel around her head, from ear to ear. If she seems unhappy or cries, place still hands on the area you are massaging to comfort her. If she settles, you can continue or try another stroke. If not, stop, wrap her in a towel, pick her up, and give her a reassuring cuddle. Resume the massage once she has relaxed, or try again the next day.

A CHILD PSYCHOLOGIST'S VIEW

DANCE OF COMMUNICATION Babies have a strong motivation to connect with people. Even when your baby is very young, she will react to your voice and your touch, so use them to communicate your feelings for her.

As she begins to recognize the things you do, she will respond to them in her own way. And as you learn to recognize her responses, and respond back, the two of you establish a "dance of communication," long before your baby uses language.

This "dance" may start with the two of you gazing at each other, then move on to smiling at each other. Slowly, your baby will begin to imitate your expressions, until

eventually, her communications become vocal and you begin to hear emerging words.

To encourage your baby's developing communication skills, keep the "dance" alive. Give her sounds, words, expressions, and caresses to respond to, and continue to return her responses. You will enjoy these "conversations" as much as your baby does, especially as her progress becomes evident.

By paying such close attention to her, you will also learn to recognize your baby's rhythms—when she likes to be calm and quiet and when she wants to be stimulated. You can then respond to her appropriately.

OLDER BABIES

❖

ONCE YOUR BABY IS ROLLING OVER, sitting up, or crawling, you will find it hard to give him a full-body massage because he will rarely lie still. Go along with this. If you still want to massage him, you must be flexible. If he rolls over from his back on to his front, for instance, massage his back. This wriggling may continue until your child is two or three.

MASSAGE, TOUCH, AND COMMUNICATION

Some older babies are happy to be massaged while sitting up. With your baby in this position, you can massage his arms (*see pages 18–19*) and back (*see pages 26–29*), and perform arm stretches (*see below*)—many babies enjoy these. If he resists massage, do not persist: he is telling you he does not want it.

MASSAGE SITTING UP

1 Sit on the floor with your baby facing you. Stretch your baby's arms straight out to the sides. Pull the arms outward gently and hold the position for a few seconds.

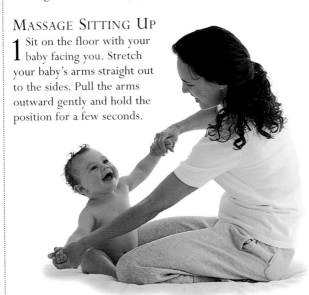

2 Cross your baby's arms over his chest, with his right arm over his left arm. Repeat step 1, then cross his arms again, this time left over right. Repeat steps 1 and 2 several times.

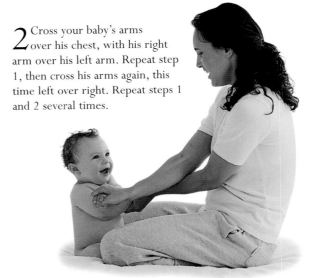

PHYSICAL CLOSENESS
Although massage is a lovely way to be physical with your baby, it is important that you do not continue if he would rather not be massaged. You can find other ways of being close to him. Sing songs or rhymes that involve actions such as bouncing him on your knee. Or you can simply cuddle him on your lap.

SEPARATION ANXIETY
Around the time that massage becomes less possible, you may notice that your child begins to experience "separation anxiety." He may cry each time you leave the room and want to be carried for long periods of time. This happens because he wants to feel secure in exploring the world and is testing his security—you. If you give him the feeling of security he needs now, it will help him to become confident and independent in time. Pick him up and take him with you if you move across or out of the room. Do not see this as a burden or a chore, but as an opportunity to be close and to help him feel safe.

COMMUNICATING THAT YOU UNDERSTAND HIS NEEDS

As your baby becomes older, he will start initiating communication. He will try to indicate to you what he does and does not like—by refusing milk or a spoonful of food, for example. Respond to his communications in a way that makes it clear that he is understood. If he shows he is not enjoying a massage stroke, try another that you know he likes. At this stage of his development, he needs to know that you can understand what he is trying to express, and can give him what he needs from you.

Your baby's needs will continue to develop, and responding to them appropriately can be a challenge. During the first eight to nine months, he needs you to be consistent and reliable, so he knows you are there for him.

A CHILD PSYCHOLOGIST'S VIEW

RESPONDING TO HIS NEEDS If you respond consistently to your baby's requirements, he will know he can rely on you to understand and meet his needs. This has a positive impact on his emotional and psychological development. A sense of security during infancy is the foundation for a healthy emotional life.

Use physical touch to let your baby know that you understand his needs, particularly if he shows anxiety about being separated from you

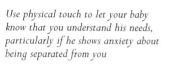

TODDLERS

❖

WHEN YOUR CHILD STARTS TO WALK, a massage routine becomes impossible; it will be difficult to get him to sit still, let alone lie still. You can reintroduce massage when your toddler is two and a half to three years old, depending on his personality. Until then, communicate with him using other touch techniques. He will love cuddles on your lap and having his hair stroked. When you talk to him, touch his arm or leg gently. Stroke his tummy or back as part of his bedtime routine, together with kisses and cuddles. Play games and sing songs that involve touch, smiles, and eye contact. You will enjoy giving him this attention as much as he loves to receive it, and he will know you love and value him.

GROWING INDEPENDENCE

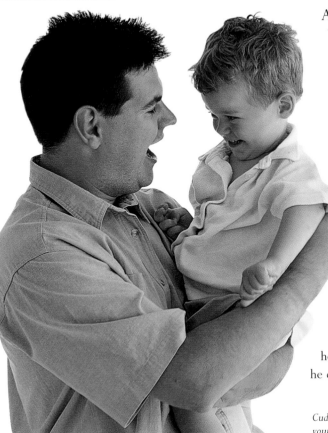

ASSERTING HIS WILL

To test his growing independence, your toddler will frequently try to assert his will. Often, parents mistake this behavior as willfulness in the adult sense, and feel they have somehow failed in their parenting. But this is not the case. It is a natural step in every child's development. However, toddlers often do not know what they want or what is best for them. That is why they need their parents to help them.

LETTING HIM CHOOSE

Even if he has enjoyed massage for many months, a toddler may suddenly decide "not today." This is fine. You have to insist on some things—a warm coat on a cold day, for instance—but massage can wait. Your toddler may allow you to massage parts of his body—his back, face or arms—until you find he is enjoying the process he initially refused. But if he continues to refuse, be sensitive to his wishes.

Cuddles, games, and eye contact are valuable ways of showing your toddler that you love him and enjoy being with him

ROUTINES AND BOUNDARIES

If your toddler lets you massage her and enjoys a certain stroke in particular, go ahead and repeat it. This shows her she can influence you, and that you notice what feels good to her. A little later in her development she may begin making demands for what she wants, using words such as "more" or "again." This is a good time to establish boundaries. Your efforts to understand and respond to your baby's needs reap rewards at this stage, since you must be able to distinguish between what she needs and what she simply wants in order not to deny your child anything essential. When appropriate, say "no," but be prepared for her to test the boundaries. For example, she may try to extend her bedtime routine by asking for "one more story." This is when parents know best—one or two stories are enough! Keeping boundaries and routines is part of good parenting—do it gently and clearly.

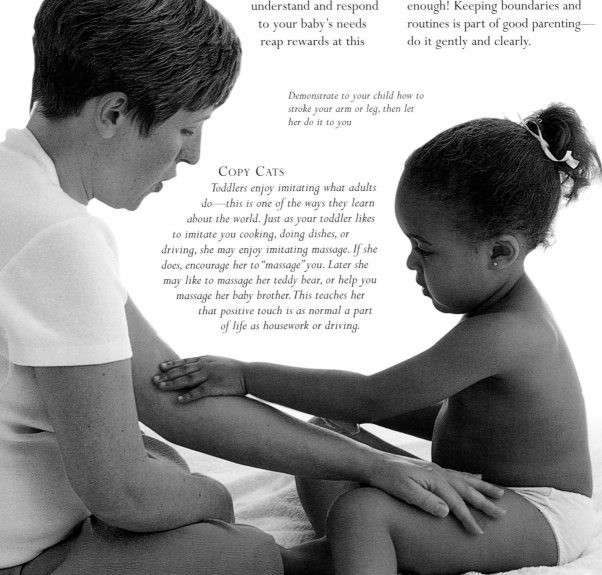

Demonstrate to your child how to stroke your arm or leg, then let her do it to you

COPY CATS

Toddlers enjoy imitating what adults do—this is one of the ways they learn about the world. Just as your toddler likes to imitate you cooking, doing dishes, or driving, she may enjoy imitating massage. If she does, encourage her to "massage" you. Later she may like to massage her teddy bear, or help you massage her baby brother. This teaches her that positive touch is as normal a part of life as housework or driving.

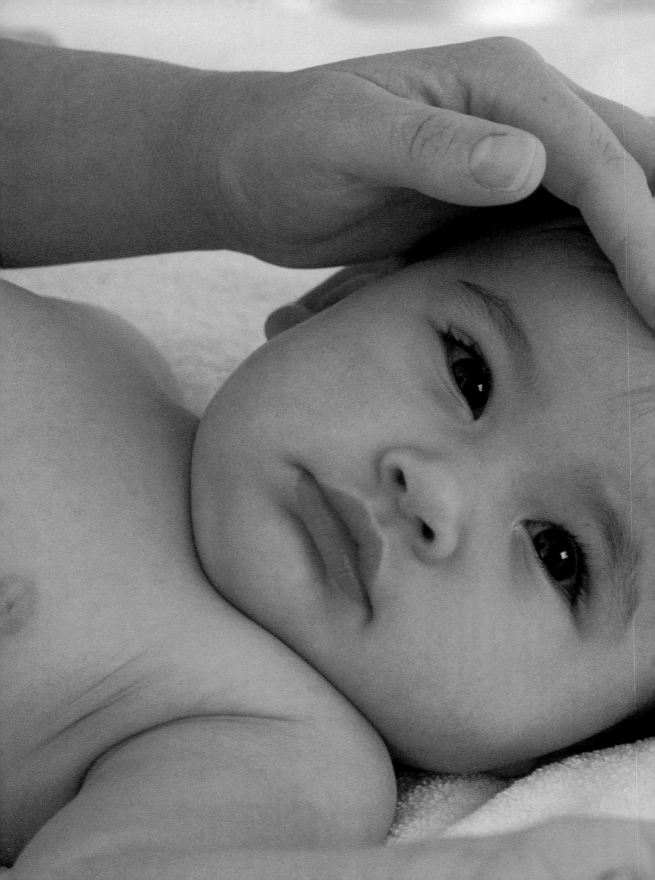

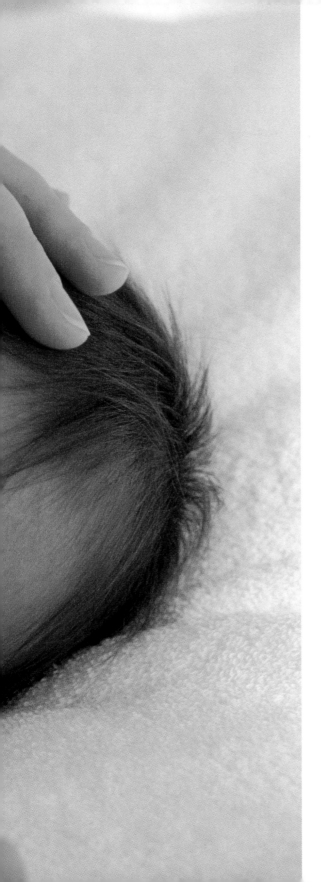

EASING COMMON PROBLEMS

---   ❖   ---

IT IS UNLIKELY THAT YOUR CHILD WILL
PASS THROUGH INFANCY AND EARLY
CHILDHOOD WITHOUT ENCOUNTERING
SOME OF THE MINOR AILMENTS, OR OTHER
SOURCES OF DISTRESS, THAT ARE COMMON
IN THESE AGE GROUPS. BABY MASSAGE
CAN HELP TO EASE THE PAIN AND
DISCOMFORT CAUSED BY SOME OF THESE
PROBLEMS, BUT EVEN WHEN IT DOES NOT,
MANY PARENTS OFTEN FIND IT WORKS
WELL AS A COPING STRATEGY WHEN A
CHILD IS SICK. IT ALLOWS YOU TO FEEL
YOU HAVE TRIED YOUR BEST TO HELP.
BABIES SENSE THIS CONCERN, AND CAN
BE COMFORTED BY IT.

---   ❖   ---

COLIC & GAS

❖

Long periods of inconsolable crying that usually last from about two weeks of age until a baby is 12 to 14 weeks old are often referred to as colic. The cause is unknown, but recent research suggests that colic may be an extreme form of normal crying. Commonly, the crying is worse in the evenings. Babies with gas often cry in pain until the gas is passed. After carrying an inconsolable baby around for hours, parents often feel helpless, exhausted, and distressed themselves. They may also feel disillusioned, since the reality of colic is far from the vision of parenthood they might have had. Certain massage strokes can help to relieve colic temporarily or expel gas. By bringing some relief to their baby, parents may also feel more able to cope with the ongoing situation.

COPING WITH COLIC AND GAS

SIGNS AND SYMPTOMS
Typically, babies with gas or colic:
❖ are difficult to burp
❖ become fretful when lying on their backs
❖ bring their knees up to their chests frequently
❖ are less distressed when held in an upright position
❖ arch backward
❖ have a distressed cry that does not stop when they are picked up, or stops only to start again.

THINGS TO TRY
Since each baby is different, techniques that relieve one baby may not work for another. You could try:
❖ holding positions (*see opposite*)
❖ carrying your baby positioned over your shoulder
❖ movement—putting your baby in a rocking baby seat or rocking him in your arms, walking him in a sling, pushing him in a stroller, or taking him for a drive
❖ giving him a deep, warm, relaxing bath; take him in the bathtub with you—this may calm you both down
❖ over-the-counter medication
❖ homeopathic remedies.

SUCKING
Babies with colic or gas like to suck because it reduces pain. It provides a distraction and also helps the body to produce endorphins, which help to relieve pain naturally. Some babies like to suck on a pacifier; others prefer their own or a parent's finger. Since sucking offers temporary relief, some parents feed their babies very frequently, especially if breastfeeding. Once breastfeeding is established, stick to one feeding every two or three hours to allow time for digestion. Cooled boiled water, from a spoon or a cup, may help to bring up gas before a feeding.

RESEARCH EVIDENCE

Research has found that colic can damage parent–baby relationships. Parents lose confidence when their efforts to soothe their colicky baby are fruitless. Because they feel inadequate, when their baby expresses a need, they respond with confusion rather than positive action. Massage can relieve colic temporarily, but it can also aid in breaking the cycle of ineffectuality, since parents feel their actions do, in some way, help their baby.

TECHNIQUES FOR PAIN RELIEF

There are various massage strokes (*see pages 80–81*) that may ease your baby's colic or help him to pass gas. Perform the strokes when he is not distressed—or at least, not too distressed. If lying on his back increases your baby's pain, place him on your lap, with his head by your knees and his feet by your hips, and raise your knees so he is lying at an angle. You can massage him with his clothes and diaper on, but you may achieve better results if he is naked. Wait for at least 30 minutes after a feeding before you massage. The holding positions shown here may also bring temporary relief to babies with colic or gas.

HOLDING POSITIONS

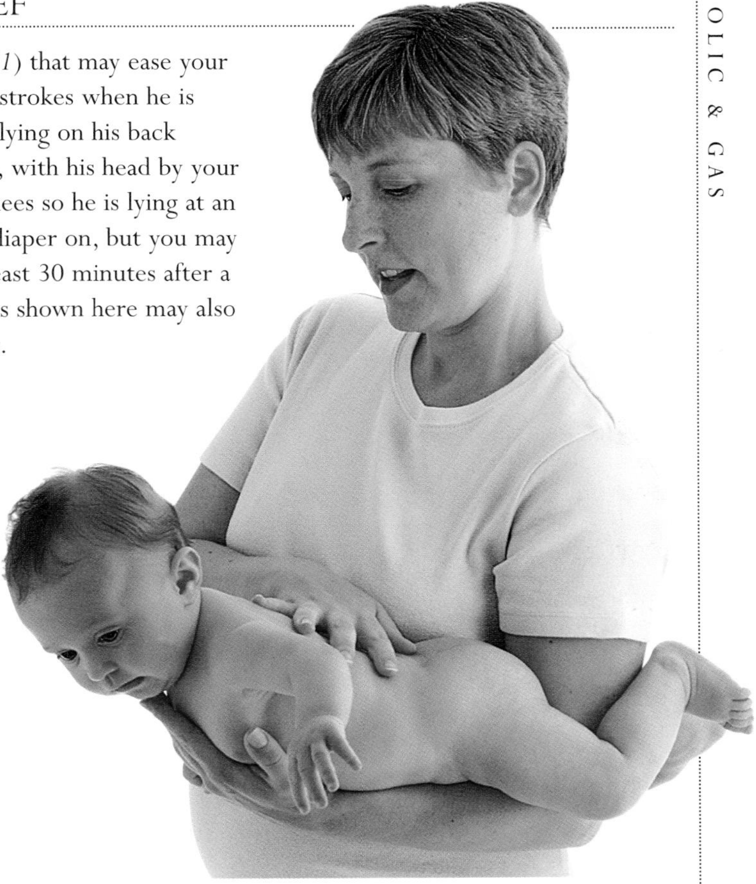

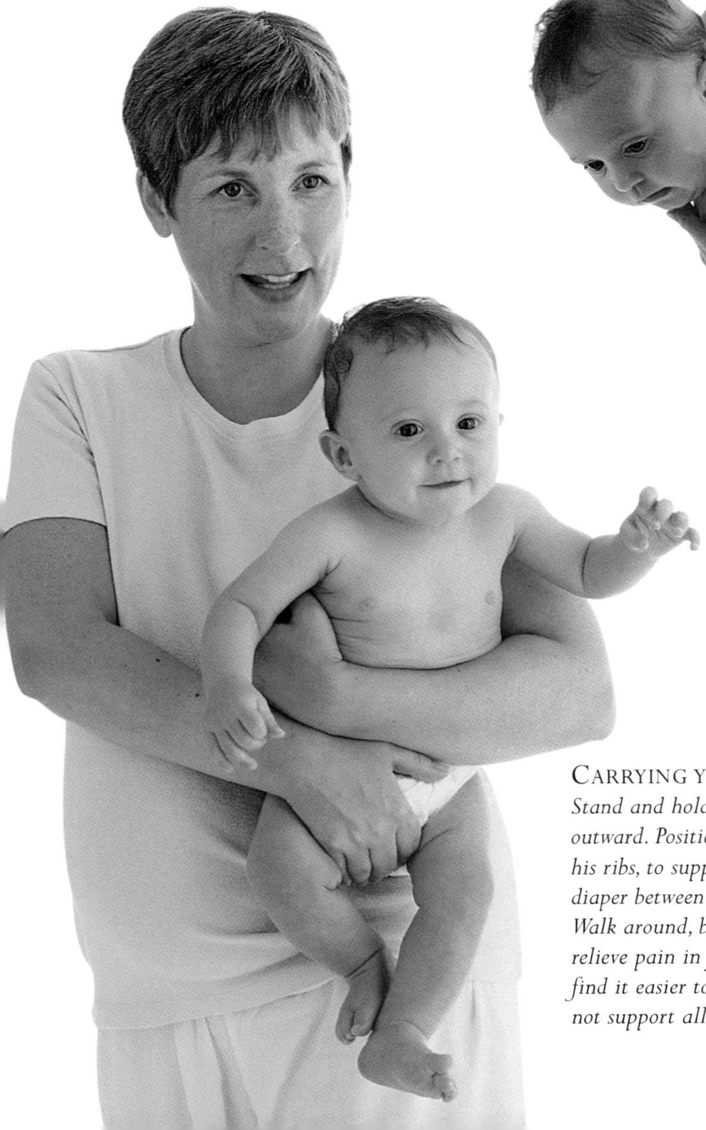

BOUNCING YOUR BABY ON YOUR ARM
Stand with one arm outstretched and place your baby on your forearm, with his head closest to your hand and his legs straddling your upper arm. Position your free hand firmly on his back to keep him steady. Press the heel of your lower hand into his abdomen, just below the ribs. Now bounce your outstretched arm up and down gently. This may relieve your baby's stomach pain and bring up gas.

CARRYING YOUR BABY UPRIGHT
Stand and hold your baby upright against your chest, facing outward. Position one arm around him across his abdomen, below his ribs, to support his weight. Place your free hand over his diaper between the front of his thighs to help keep him balanced. Walk around, bouncing gently, or bounce in place. This may relieve pain in your baby's abdomen and bring up gas. You may find it easier to position his bottom on your hip so your arm does not support all his weight.

STROKES TO EASE COLIC AND GAS

1 ▼MASSAGING THE SIDES OF THE ABDOMEN Position your baby on his back with his feet closest to you. Place your hand on one side of his abdomen, fingers pointing downward. Pull the flesh up toward the navel, then repeat the stroke with your other hand. Continue in this way, using both hands consecutively in a rhythmic action, then repeat on his other side. This helps to empty the stomach of its contents.

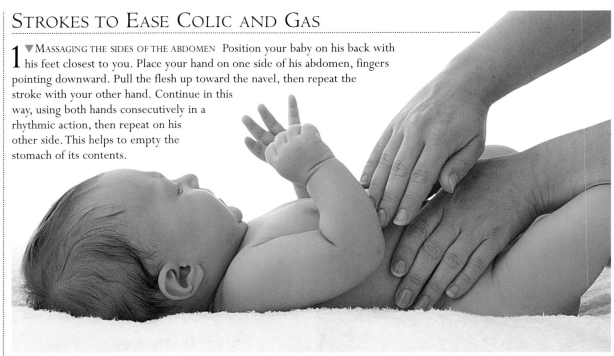

2 LITTLE CIRCLES AROUND THE NAVEL Hold the first two fingers of one hand together and place them next to your baby's navel. Press gently, making a circular motion, then release the pressure. Slide your fingers an inch or so clockwise around the navel and repeat. Continue in this way, spiraling outward until you reach the inside of your baby's right hip (*see page 21*). This stroke moves the contents of the small intestine. Working in a clockwise direction follows the natural flow of the digestive tract.

3 LARGE CIRCLES AROUND THE ABDOMEN Place your hand on your baby's abdomen, just inside his right hip. Stroke up firmly with the flat of your fingers and your palm until you reach the right side of the rib cage. Leading with your fingers, stroke across the diaphragm to the same point on your baby's left side. Now stroke down to just inside his left hip, then across the base of the abdomen to the starting position (*see page 21*). Repeat several times. This stroke encourages the contents of the colon to move forward.

4 ▼CYCLING MOVEMENTS WITH THE LEGS Hold your baby's ankles and bend one knee up to his abdomen, then straighten the leg. As you gently pull it straight, bend his other knee up to his abdomen. Repeat this "cycling" movement slowly and rhythmically a few times. This motion can help your baby to expel gas.

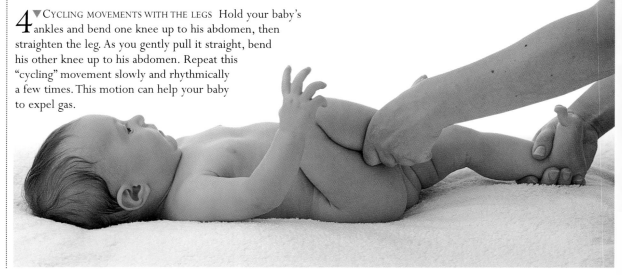

5 BENDING THE KNEES SIMULTANEOUSLY Take hold of your baby's ankles, one in each hand. Bend both his legs to bring his knees up to his abdomen. Hold his legs in this position for a few seconds, then straighten them gently. Repeat slowly several times. This action may help to relieve abdominal pain caused by gas.

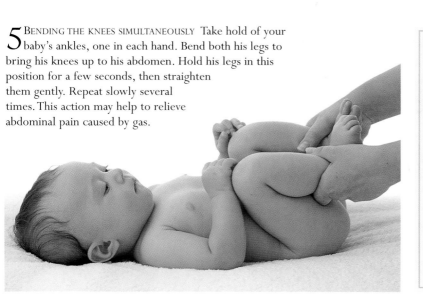

6 MASSAGING THE BASE OF THE SPINE Turn your baby over to lie on his front, with his feet closest to you. Place the heel of your hand in the dimple just above the center of his buttocks. Move the heel of your hand in a clockwise direction, pressing gently. Repeat several times. This stroke helps your baby to expel gas.

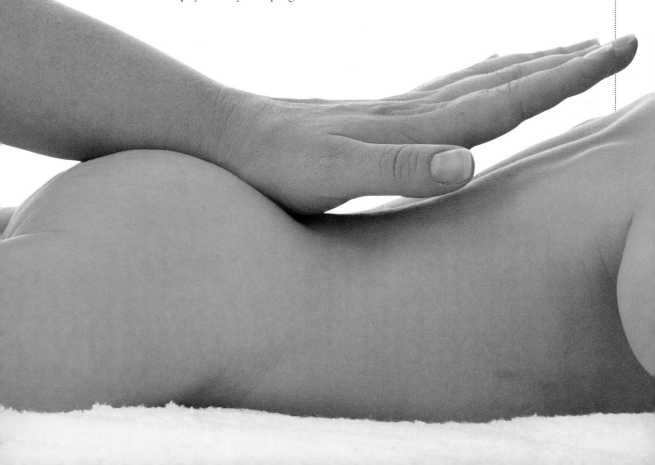

CONSTIPATION

❖

FROM TIME TO TIME, your baby may suffer from constipation. Massaging her abdominal area can be an effective way of both relieving and preventing this. The massage can be done when she is fully clothed, but is more effective if she is naked. Allow at least one hour after a feeding before performing the strokes shown here. For this massage sequence, lay your baby on her back with her feet closest to you.

COPING WITH CONSTIPATION

SIGNS AND SYMPTOMS

❖ NO STOOLS

A constipated child will frequently strain to pass a stool, but does not always achieve it.

❖ HARD STOOLS

When a stool is passed, it is hard, often resembling a solid pellet.

❖ CRYING

A hard stool can be painful to pass, so babies often cry just before and while passing a stool.

❖ TIME LAPSE BETWEEN STOOLS

If your child has not passed a stool for over three days, it is possible that she is constipated. It is normal for babies and young children to pass stools three times a day, and also normal not to "go" at all for up to three days, and sometimes even longer if they are being breast-fed.

❖ STRAINING

Although it is a sign of constipation, "straining" is not always a reliable indicator—babies often get red in the face when pushing out a stool. If your child strains when passing a stool, then passes a soft, well-formed one, she is not constipated.

THINGS TO TRY

Besides abdominal massage, there are other options you should consider to relieve constipation or to prevent it from occurring:

❖ PLENTY OF FLUIDS

Make sure your baby is drinking enough fluids. Freshly squeezed orange juice can help to move the bowels. Give your child two to four fluid ounces of diluted orange juice a day. Squeeze some oranges, strain the juice, and dilute it to a ratio of one part orange juice to four parts boiled and cooled water.

❖ A HEALTHY DIET

Does your baby's diet include all she needs to prevent constipation? Up to four months, she should have breast or formula milk and juices. From four months, give her baby cereal, cornmeal, pureed fruits and vegetables, and stewed dried fruit. From six months, introduce cereals, legumes, and other grains gradually. Fiber and fluids help prevent constipation, but do not omit fat from the diet. Ask your doctor for advice if necessary.

❖ SENSIBLE ADVICE

Constipation can be a common problem with babies and young children. If it occurs, it tends to be recurring. Your doctor or pediatrician will be able to give you useful advice and support in coping with a constipated baby.

CASE HISTORY

"Rhian first became constipated when she started on solids. I tried giving her diluted orange juice as well as breastfeedings, and stewed prunes and apricots, but nothing seemed to help. I found it very upsetting seeing her straining so much. Sometimes she did not pass a stool for six or seven days. My sister massaged her children and offered to show me some strokes on the tummy that she felt might help. Amazingly, it worked! I would massage Rhian's tummy and then, when she started to strain, bend her knees up to her tummy and bring them back down again. I now use the massage each time Rhian is constipated, and also regularly to try to prevent it."

STROKES TO EASE CONSTIPATION

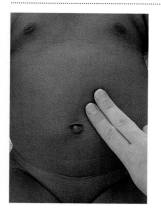

1 LITTLE CIRCLES AROUND THE NAVEL Place the first two fingers of one hand next to the navel. Press gently, making a circular motion, and release. Slide the fingers around the navel slightly and repeat. Work clockwise, spiraling outward to the right hip. This follows the flow of the small intestine, moving its contents along the digestive tract.

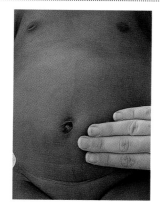

2 LARGE CIRCLES AROUND THE ABDOMEN Starting just inside the right hip, move your flat fingers and palm up to the right side of the rib cage, then across to the same point on the left side. Stroke down to just inside the left hip, then along the base of the abdomen to the right hip. Repeat several times. This shifts the contents of the colon.

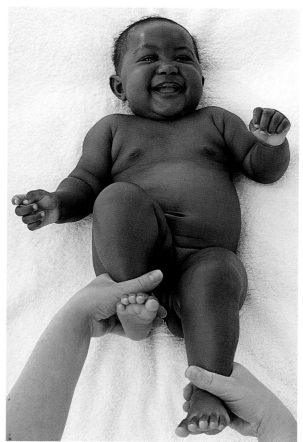

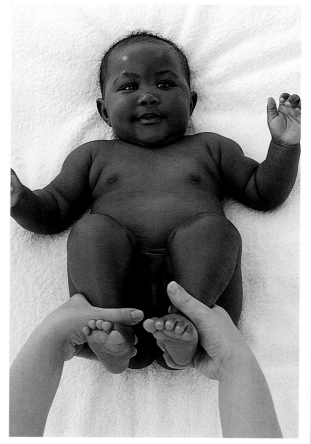

3 CYCLING MOVEMENTS WITH THE LEGS Hold your baby's ankles and bend one knee, bringing it up toward her abdomen. Now pull the leg gently until it is straight, and bend her other knee up to the abdomen as before. Repeat this "cycling" motion slowly and rhythmically several times. This action may encourage a bowel movement.

4 BENDING THE KNEES SIMULTANEOUSLY Hold your baby's ankles and bend both her knees at the same time, bringing them up toward her abdomen. Hold her legs in this position for a few seconds, then pull them down gently until they are straight. Repeat slowly a number of times. This technique can help to open your baby's bowels.

FUSSY CRYING

❖

BABIES CRY ON AVERAGE for two hours in every 24. Often, the cause of distress is obvious and easily remedied, but at other times, it can be unclear. Whatever the reason, if your baby cries, pick him up and cuddle him. The results of research studies indicate that the quicker a parent responds to a crying baby, the sooner the child stops crying. In some cases, nothing soothes screaming babies, which can be very frustrating for parents. Massage may calm your crying baby, but even if it does not, you could find that, between bouts of crying, both you and your baby enjoy massage and are relaxed by it.

COPING WITH A CRYING BABY

REASONS FOR DISTRESS
Typically, babies cry because they:
❖ are hungry
❖ need a diaper change
❖ want to be cuddled
❖ are tired and need to sleep
❖ want a change of position
❖ are overstimulated
❖ feel pain or are uncomfortable.

THINGS TO TRY
❖ PHYSICAL CLOSENESS
Babies may be soothed by cuddling. Sing to your baby while holding him. You may feel it is wrong for your baby to fall asleep in your arms. Do not worry about this—responding to his needs is more important.
❖ MOTION
Walk your baby around the house in your arms or a sling. Push him in a stroller or take him for a car ride.
❖ DISTRACTIONS
Try distracting your baby with a mobile, a musical toy, or a peek at the world through the window.

❖ BATHING
Water can be soothing, so try giving your baby a bath.
❖ HANDING HIM OVER
If you are tense, your baby may sense this and cry more. He may relax if he is held by someone else, which also gives you a chance to rest.
❖ SWADDLING
Being contained can make babies feel secure. It is important that his arms are bent, with hands placed up by the mouth so he can self-soothe by sucking his fingers.

INCONSOLABLE BABIES
If your baby cries for long periods, and you do not know why, your confidence may be undermined and you may feel upset, frustrated, and tired. If you feel angry with your baby for crying, or overwhelmed, put him in a safe place, such as his crib, and take a few minutes away to calm down. Contact your doctor or pediatrician for advice.

RESEARCH EVIDENCE
Some parents may feel it is wrong to respond to a baby each time he cries because this might "spoil" him and give him unrealistic expectations of life. Recent research suggests that this point of view is counterproductive. The results of one study state that crying babies are soothed when lifted on to a caregiver's shoulder, and that they also become visually alert, showing that this attention is nurturing. Investigation into child psychology has established that by responding to a baby's needs, parents actually help to build his confidence (see pages 72–73). Nature also supports these theories: the same study reports that mothers are naturally compelled to attend to their crying babies and to stay close until they are calm. The study also found that mothers can distinguish a "pain" cry from a less serious one. And it is also true that most adults want to "do something" about a crying baby.

MASSAGE FOR FUSSY BABIES

If your baby is accustomed to massage, you may be able to use it to help him calm down when he is crying. If he has not been massaged before, massage him a few times between bouts of crying to familiarize him with the strokes. Try using the strokes that you know he usually enjoys most of all. Effleurage strokes are soothing and reassuring because they are long, firm, and rhythmic. The strokes shown below concentrate on the abdomen and back of the baby, but you can also try effleurage strokes on the front and back of the legs (see pages 22 and 31), as well as on the arms (see page 18). If your baby continues to cry, stop the massage, wrap him in a towel to keep him warm, and pick him up. You may be able to massage him between bouts of crying, but do not try it if he becomes distressed.

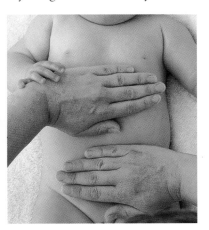

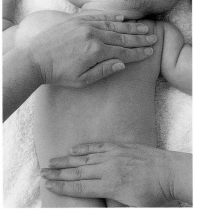

Hold your baby to comfort him when he is crying, and try to distract him from his distress by singing a song or showing him a toy or colorful object

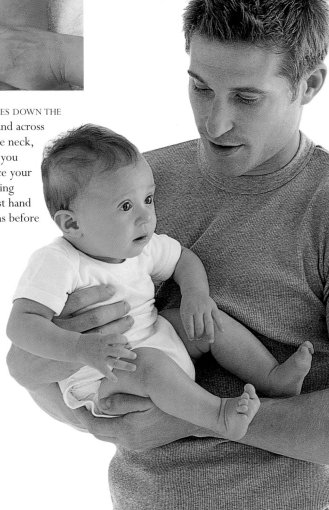

1 EFFLEURAGE STROKES DOWN THE ABDOMEN Position one hand across the abdomen, below the chest. Stroke down to the base of the abdomen, placing your other hand in the starting position as you do so. Just before the first hand lifts off, begin the stroke as before with the other. Repeat several times, with one hand always in contact with your baby's body.

2 EFFLEURAGE STROKES DOWN THE BACK Place one hand across the back, just below the neck, and stroke down until you reach the bottom. Place your other hand in the starting position before the first hand lifts off. Stroke down as before with the second hand. Repeat several times.

CASE HISTORY

"I took Laura to the clinic at four weeks. She had been crying almost continuously since she was two days old. By this time I was exhausted (she wasn't sleeping much) and at the end of my rope. An expert in baby massage came to see us at home. When Laura wasn't crying, she showed me how to perform a full-body massage on her. I saw right away that Laura loved it. Now I massage her a few times a week, and when she cries—it usually calms her down. She is much happier these days, and sleeps better. I think the massage really helped her."

TEETHING

❖

MOST BABIES EXPERIENCE pain or discomfort when their teeth come through, as their gums become swollen. Massage helps because pressure can soothe swollen gums. The strokes shown here may ease your baby's teething pain temporarily, and encourage him to relax if he is fretful. Practice these strokes before teething begins, if possible, so that your baby is familiar with them and will allow you to perform them on him when his gums are uncomfortable. Also, try performing a full-body massage on your baby: this stimulates the production of endorphins in his body, which may help to alleviate pain.

RECOGNIZING TEETHING

SIGNS AND SYMPTOMS

Babies who are teething may:
❖ chew their fingers, or put them in their mouths
❖ have red cheeks
❖ have a fever
❖ suffer from red or inflamed gums
❖ have red skin in the diaper area.

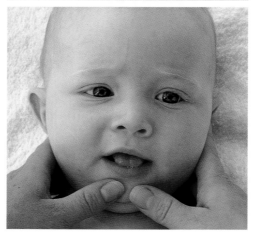

CASE HISTORY

"I took Rebecca to baby-massage classes when she was six weeks old. A couple of the strokes the teacher showed us involved pressing the gums through the skin, above and below the lips. She said these strokes might ease teething pain. When Rebecca began teething, I tried those strokes. She enjoyed them and stopped being crabby for a while afterward, smiling and laughing again. I think they distracted her from the pain."

1 CIRCLES ON THE UPPER GUM LINE Place your thumbs next to each other on the dip above the top lip. Press gently with each thumb, making a small, circular motion, then release the pressure. Move your thumbs outward a little and repeat. Do this along the length of the upper lip, continuing along the top jawline to the sides of the ears.

2 CIRCLES ON THE LOWER GUM LINE Position your thumbs next to each other just below the center of your baby's lower lip. Press gently, making small circular movements with your thumb, then release. Slide your thumbs outward a little way and repeat. Work along the length of the gum line in this way, then continue along the lower jawline and up to the sides of the ears.

DRY SKIN

❖

SOMETIMES BABIES ARE BORN with dry, flaky skin on the face, hands, feet, or all over the body. In other cases, patches of dry skin develop over time, typically on the elbows, upper arms, diaper area, or between the eyebrows. Regular oiling usually clears the problem, and by massaging the oil in, you allow it to penetrate the skin deeply. Use a natural oil such as sunflower oil. Rub it into the affected area once or twice a day. If you oil your baby's face, avoid the area around the eyes. Consult your doctor if the dry skin does not clear within a few days, or if it becomes red, inflamed, or worse in any way.

OILING YOUR CHILD'S SKIN

Olive, sunflower, or grapeseed oil is good for dry skin. Place some on your hands, rub them together, and glide them over the affected area. Avoid oils that contain nut products, especially if there is a history of nut allergy in your family. Dry skin may indicate sensitive skin, so watch for reactions to lotions, soaps, and detergents, and switch to an enzyme-free detergent.

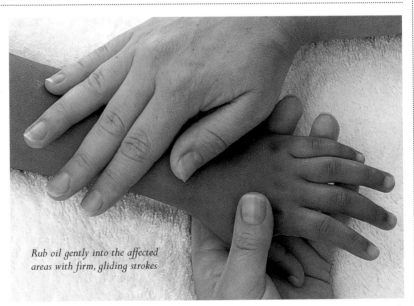

Rub oil gently into the affected areas with firm, gliding strokes

CASE HISTORY

"Daniel was a little overdue. When he was born, he had very dry skin all over his face and body. I was surprised at how scaly his skin was. My daughter also had dry skin when she was born, but not nearly as bad as Daniel's. I rubbed sunflower oil into his skin twice daily from when he was a few days old. I had already massaged my daughter, so I knew oil was good for dry skin. Daniel's skin soon became soft and velvety."

CRADLE CAP AND ECZEMA

Massaging a natural oil into the skin can relieve dry-skin conditions such as eczema and cradle cap. With cradle cap, massage a natural oil into the scalp daily, allowing the skin to absorb the oil. The dry skin eventually lifts away from the scalp. Brush it gently with your fingers, or run a comb through your baby's hair to release loosened dry skin. If your baby has eczema, massage oil into her skin to moisturize it. Do not massage the skin if it is broken, cracked, inflamed, or very red. If you suspect your child has eczema, seek medical advice.

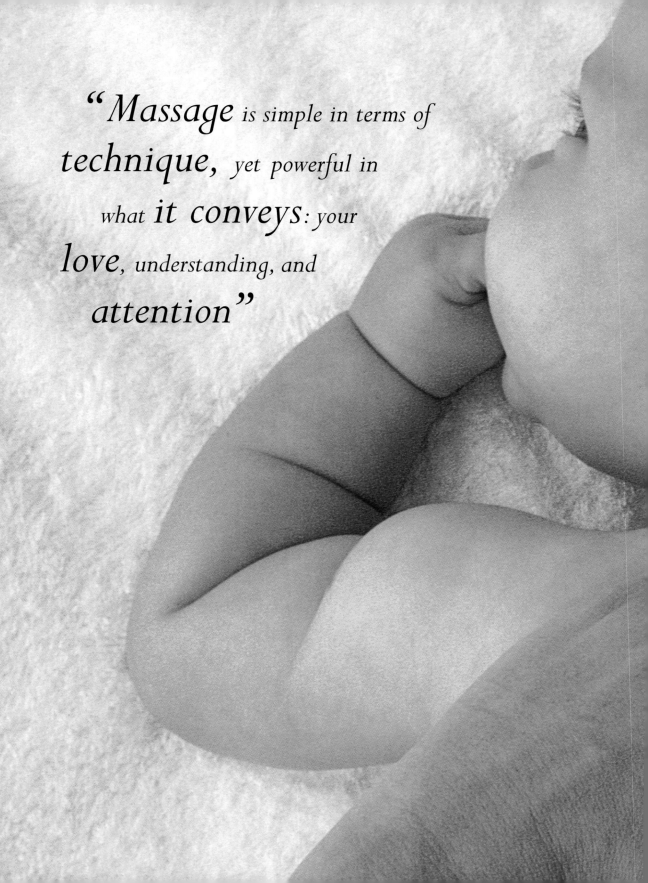

"*Massage* is simple in terms of **technique,** *yet powerful in* what **it conveys**: *your* *love*, *understanding, and* **attention**"

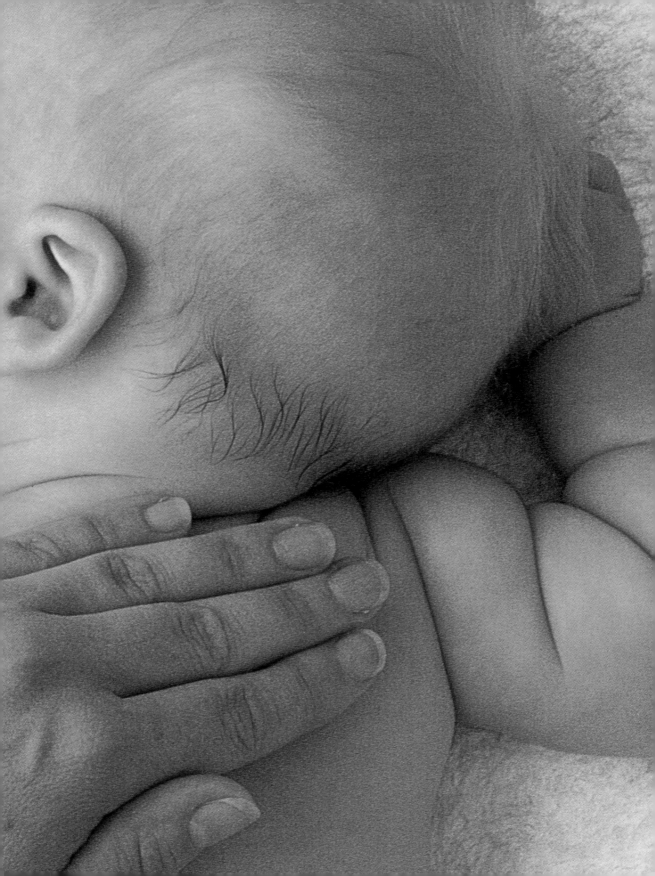

QUESTIONS & ANSWERS

❖

Q *Can I massage my baby when he has his clothes on?*

A Yes, particularly if he is newborn and if you feel both of you would like to be introduced to the massage strokes slowly. But do try to progress to removing his clothes. Children gain from any positive touch, but skin-to-skin contact—with your bare hands against your baby's skin—is the most beneficial.

Q *Should I continue to massage my baby if he has a cold or fever?*

A Avoid massaging your child if he has a fever or cold. Many children do not want a massage when they're sick, but enjoy lots of reassuring strokes and cuddles.

Q *If my child has a cut or a bruise, should I stop massaging her?*

A Avoid the bruised or cut area, which may be sore and painful to the touch. If your baby has a scar, do not massage the area until the scar has healed. But do continue to massage other areas of her body.

Q *My baby has eczema. Can I massage him?*

A Yes, you can. Use a natural oil, such as olive or sunflower oil, to moisturize your baby's skin. Choose organic oil if possible. If his skin is cracked or broken, do not massage the area until it has healed.

Q *Is massage recommended for asthmatic children?*

A An asthmatic child can benefit from massage, especially if the condition is stress- or anxiety-related. Massage may help her to relax, which could prevent asthma attacks or reduce their severity. Never massage your child during an attack, but do give her reassuring strokes on her arms, legs, or head to help her feel less frightened.

Q *Can I use essential oils to massage my baby?*

A It is not advisable to use essential oils on babies or young children. Few essential oils are suitable, and those that are should be diluted in a base oil. Never use any essential oil on your child unless instructed by a trained aromatherapist.

Q *My child has very sensitive skin and is allergic to detergents and soaps. Is it safe to use oil? What type of oil should I use?*

A A natural oil is less likely to irritate sensitive skin than a synthetic variety. Select a light oil such as sunflower or apricot, choosing an organic variety if available. The more naturally the oil is produced, the better. Before using any oil, make sure you carry out a patch test on your child (*see page 15*) to make sure she is not sensitive to the oil you choose.

Q *My baby is allergic to nuts. Will she be affected if I massage her with a nut oil?*

A Do not use a nut oil under any circumstances because it may well affect your child. Try a natural oil such as grapeseed or olive oil. Some vegetable oils may contain nut products, so before using any oil, make absolutely certain that it is free of these. If the ingredients label is unclear, contact the manufacturer for further information. Once you have chosen an oil, make sure you perform a patch test on your baby (*see page 15*) to eliminate the possibility of sensitivity. If you have any doubts, massage your baby without oil—it is the loving touch you give her that is most important.

Q *My baby has recently had surgery. Is it safe to massage her?*

A Check with your surgeon before massaging your baby postoperatively. In many cases, once a child has recovered from surgery, massage is very beneficial to the baby and her parents. The touch is soothing to the child, and massaging their baby helps parents overcome anxieties about handling an infant in a delicate state. Avoid massaging the general area of the operation until the scar has healed—your doctor can give you more advice on this.

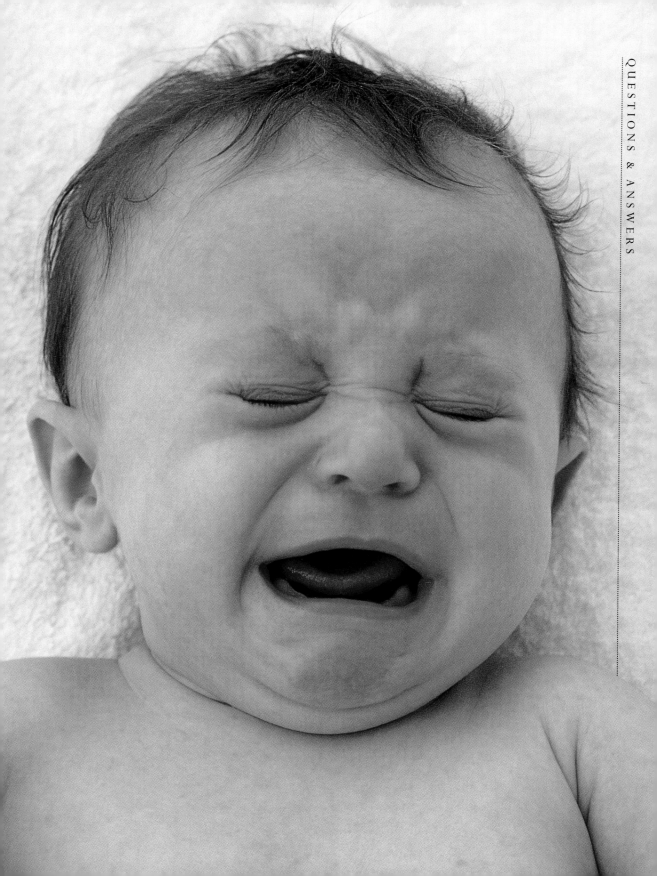

QUESTIONS & ANSWERS

❖

Q *My baby often falls asleep when I massage her. Is this bad?*

A Some babies do fall asleep during massage, especially if snuggled up to their parent. This is fine until your baby is about four months old, after which time you should help her fall asleep with less and less physical contact, so she can put herself back to sleep when she wakes up in the night. If she is accustomed to falling asleep during massage, she is unlikely to go back to sleep alone.

Q *How can I tell if I'm using the right or wrong pressure for my massage strokes?*

A Your baby's skin will redden if the pressure is too firm. This is obvious on fair-skinned children, but be aware that it is less obvious on dark skin. If your child cries, pulls away, or seems uncomfortable when you massage her, it may be that you are using too much pressure. Be aware of using too little pressure—this will give your child a tickling sensation. If you are unsure, use the pressure you would apply to rub cream into your face.

Q *I have just had a Cesarean. When can I start massaging my baby?*

A As soon as you feel you are able to. It may be hard to find a comfortable sitting position for massage, so keep the sessions short until your scar has healed.

Q *I have a bad back and find the massage positions on the floor uncomfortable. What should I do?*

A Your back pains may be caused by incorrect posture. When sitting on the floor, be sure to keep your back straight and bend forward from the hips. Sitting on more cushions may help you to do this. If the floor is still too uncomfortable, sit on a chair with a towel across your lap and your baby on the towel. Always keep one hand on your baby so she does not roll or slip off your lap. However, this position will not be safe once she is moving or rolling over, or is too big for your lap.

Q *When I massage my young baby, my toddler becomes jealous. What can I do about this?*

A It is not unusual for a toddler to be jealous of a young sibling, especially if physical contact is involved. If your toddler would like to be massaged herself, make a regular time for it, when your baby is asleep or settled, so she feels she gets the same special attention from you as your baby does. Or ask her if she would like to "help" you massage the baby. Show her how to rub oil gently into the baby's arms and legs, then praise her for doing it well. Perhaps she would enjoy massaging "her baby"—a favorite teddy bear or doll—while you massage yours.

Q *I recently adopted a toddler. Can massage help us to bond?*

A Massage may certainly be one of the ways in which you establish a bond between you and your child. Before you begin, you must familiarize yourself with what the toddler does and does not like. Some children do not like to be touched, particularly by people they do not know well. Be warm, open, and approachable. When he comes to you by himself, you will know that he is comfortable being close to you. At this point, start to touch him more and more. Stroke his hair, and put your hand on his shoulder or an arm around him when you talk to him, especially if you are telling him what a good boy he is. Start to massage him when you feel confident that he can relax and enjoy it.

Q *My child is close to the end of her toddlerhood. Is there an age when I should stop massaging her?*

A The time to stop massaging your child is when she gives you the cue. If she seems to be losing interest and often wriggles, sits up, rolls over, or walks away during massage, or if she cries or asks you not to do it, then respect her wishes and stop. If she continues to enjoy it, massage her for as long as you like, even into adulthood— it can be a special time of closeness between you then, too.

92

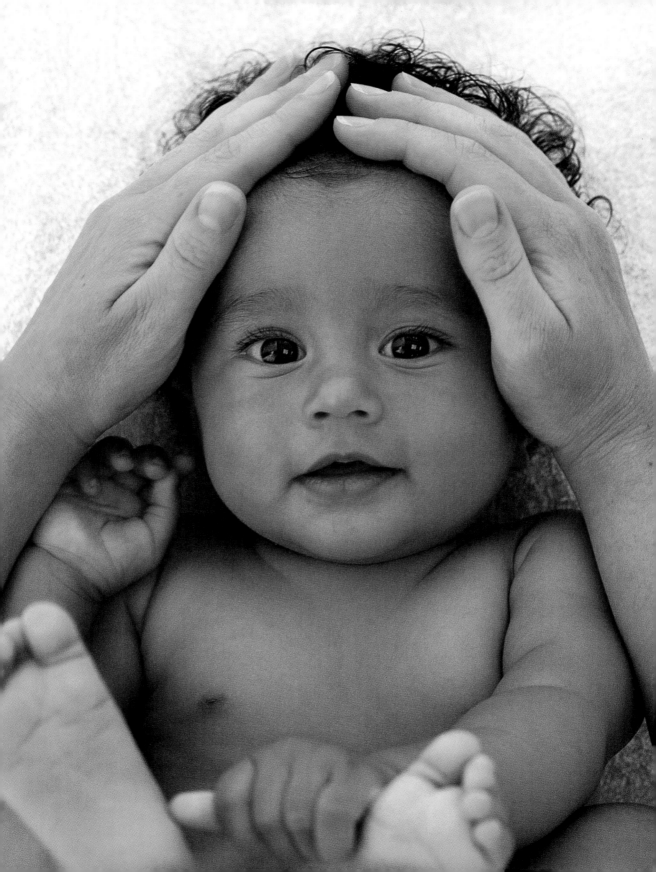

INDEX

❖

RESOURCES AND USEFUL ADDRESSES

As the benefits of infant massage become increasingly obvious, courses that teach these techniques will become more common. Your doctor or pediatrician or your local library will have a list of groups, clinics, and centers that can advise you on infant massage and tell you about the classes that are taught in your area. In some cases, information may be available through your childbirth instructor as well.

American Massage Therapy
Association
820 Davis Street
Suite 100
Evanston, IL 60201-4444
(847) 864-0123
www.amtamassage.org

Babies Today
http://babiestoday.com

International Association of Infant
Massage
1891 Goodyear Avenue
Suite 622
Ventura, CA 93003
(800) 248-5432
www.iaim-us.com

International Loving Touch
Foundation, Inc.
P.O. Box 16374
Portland, OR 97292
(503) 253-8482
www.lovingtouch.com

National Network for Child Care
Cooperative Extension System
US Department of Agriculture
www.nncc.org
Information, referrals, newsletter

Touch Research Institute
Department of Pediatrics
University of Miami
School of Medicine
1601 NW 12th Avenue
Miami, FL 33101
(305) 243-6781
www.miami.edu/touch-research
Research, information, newsletter

Canadian Massage Therapist
Alliance
344 Lakeshore Road East
Suite B
Oakville
ON L6J 1J6
(905) 849-7606
www.cmta.ca
Links to registered massage therapists
across the country

REFERENCES

page 12
"...babies who are touched lovingly become ill and cry less often than those who are not."
Informed by
❖ G.S. Liptak et al., "Enhancing Infants' Development and Parent-Practitioner Interaction with Brazelton Neonatal Assessment Scale," **Pediatric**, July 1987, vol. 72, no. 1, p. 71–78.
❖ E.S. Haris et al., "Quality of Mother–Infant Attachment and Pediatric Health Care Use," **Pediatric**, August 1989, vol. 84, no. 2, p. 248–54.
❖ D. Iwaniec et al., "Helping Emotionally Abused Children who Fail to Thrive," **Early Prediction and Prevention of Child Abuse**, edited by K. Brown et al., Wyley & Sons, 1991.
❖ S.K. Dihigo, "New Strategies for the Treatment of Colic: Modifying the Parent/Infant Interaction," **The Journal of Pediatric Health Care**, 1998, vol. 12, no. 5, p. 256–62.
"A research study was carried out...with fathers and their babies..."
Informed by
❖ K. Scholz & C.A. Samuels, "Neonatal Bathing and Massage Intervention with Fathers, Behavioural Effects 12 Weeks after Birth of the First Baby: The Sunraysia Australia Intervention Project," **International Journal of Behavioural Development**, 1992, vol.15, no.3, p. 67–81.

page 45
"...positive touch given in addition to routine handling..."
Informed by
❖ E. Lozoff et al., "The Mother–Newborn Relationship: Limits of Adaptability," **The Journal of Pediatrics**, July 1997, vol. 99, no. 1, p. 1–12.
❖ L. Casler, "The Effects of Extra-Tactile Stimulation of a Group of Institutionalised Infants," **Genealogy and Psychological Monograph**, 1965, vol. 71, p. 137–75. Cited in G. Westland (1993), "Massage as a Therapeutic Tool: Part 1," **British Journal of Occupational Therapy**, vol. 56, no. 4, p. 129–34.

page 62
"A research study was conducted in 1995..."
Informed by
❖ Lynda Harrison, Linda Olivet, Kathy Cunningham, Mary Beth Bodin and Cindy Hicks, "Effects of Gentle Human Touch on Preterm Infants: Pilot Study Results," **Neonatal Network**, March 1996, vol. 15, no.2, p. 35–42.
❖ D. Nelson et al., "Effects of Tactile Stimulation on Premature Infant Weight Gain," **Journal of Obstetric, Gynaecological and Neonatal Nursing**, May/June 1986, p. 262–67.
❖ T. Field et al., "Massage of Preterm Newborns to Improve Growth and Development," **Pediatric Nursing**, November/December 1987, vol. 1, no. 6, p. 385–87.
❖ R.C. White-Traut & M.B. Goldman, "Premature Infant Massage—Is It Safe?," **Pediatric Nursing**, 1988, vol. 14, no. 4, p. 285–89

❖ L. Paterson, "Baby Massage on the Neonatal Unit," **Nursing**, December 1990, vol. 4, no. 3, p. 19–21.

page 78
"...colic can damage parent–baby relationships."
Informed by
❖ S.K. Dihigo, "New Strategies for the Treatment of Colic: Modifying the Parent/Infant Interaction," **The Journal of Pediatric Health Care**, 1998, vol. 12, no. 5, p. 256–62.

page 84
"...the quicker a parent responds to a crying baby..."
Informed by
❖ E. Lozoff et al., "The Mother-Newborn Relationship: Limits of Adaptability," **The Journal of Pediatrics**, July 1997, vol. 99, no. 1, p. 1–12.
"...this point of view is counterproductive."
Informed by
❖ I. St. James-Roberts et al., "Stability and Outcome of Persistent Infant Crying," **Infant Behaviour and Development**, 1998, vol. 21, no. 3, p. 411–35.
"...crying babies are soothed when lifted on to a caregiver's shoulder....mothers are naturally compelled to attend to their crying babies... mothers can distinguish a pain cry..."
Informed by
❖ E. Lozoff et al., "The Mother–Newborn Relationship: Limits of Adaptability," **The Journal of Pediatrics**, July 1997, vol. 99, no. 1, p. 1–12.

ACKNOWLEDGMENTS

AUTHORS' ACKNOWLEDGMENTS
Nicki Bainbridge: I would like to thank Alan Heath; Sonia Prazeres, my baby-massage teacher; Jane Scofield, Meena Davis and Mary Magowan of Community Health South London; my clients, who have taught me much; my mother Rosemary Bainbridge for her faith in me, her enthusiasm and encouragement; my husband Richard Hatton for his love, support, and flexibility; my children Daisy and Edward for their amenability while I wrote this book, and for teaching me so much about massage and touch; Ruth Bryan, Barbara and Graham Hatton for their help with child care; the team at Dorling Kindersley and all those who worked on the photo shoots, including Julie Fisher, whose fun, calm, and relaxed manner resulted in beautiful pictures.
Alan Heath: For their help, support, patience, guidance, and advice, I would like to thank Drs. Eve Rossor, Gill duMont, and Aideen Naughton, and Annie Humphris, Jane Thorpe, Janet Abbot, Christine Prior, Geraldine Finney, and Jane Schofield.

PUBLISHER'S ACKNOWLEDGMENTS
Dorling Kindersley would like to thank Nicola Cox and Conrad van Dyk for DTP design work, Sue Carlton for the index, Clare Hacking for proofreading, Mark Weyman, and Habitat and PHP (Perfectly Happy People) for providing props.
Models Melanie and Jason Ashenden, Robina Aslam and Sophia Maria O'Reilly, Nicki Bainbridge, Georgie Caine, Allen and Tanis Clarke, Ziz and Zoe Chater, Carey Combe and Cordelia Hawkins, Arden Devine, Mysanwy and Chen Dew, Lee-Ann and Amirah Edwards, Thor and Jasper Haley, Donna Harding and Star Epiphany, Margarita Foncenada and Gabriella Grant-Foncenada, Lisa Greenspan and Silas Parker, Ophelia Jackson, Michele, Kamilah and Tariq Jogee, Jeremy, Spencer and Ellis Roots, Isobel Stewart, Claire Trotman and Jasmine Graham, Jackie Vanhorne and Shannon Vanhorne-Quartey, Tomos Vaughan-Streater and Johnathan Ward.
Makeup Artists Amanda Clarke and Elizabeth Burridge.
Additional Photography p. 6, 50, 66, 76, Liz McAulay.